The Plane Always Leaves

A Visiting Forensic Psychiatrist on Circuit in the Arctic

AG Ahmed MD

The Plane Always Leaves

ISBN: 978-1-969978-95-1

Dedication

For the people of the North—
those who live with the consequences long after the plane leaves,
and those who remain to hold care, dignity, and justice together between flights.

Acknowledgements

To the communities of the North who welcomed a visitor into spaces of profound vulnerability and responsibility, thank you for the trust, the patience, and the corrections that made my work safer and more accurate.

To the local nurses, mental health workers, community wellness teams, and clinic staff who carried the daily continuity that my visits could never provide, your skill is the true infrastructure of care.

To court workers, victim services staff, interpreters, probation officers, and corrections staff, thank you for the invisible work: de-escalation, dignity, transport, translation, and the thousand tasks that keep people safe.

To colleagues in forensic psychiatry and northern health who offered mentorship, peer review, and ethical guidance, thank you for keeping rigor and humility in balance.

To my family and loved ones, who accepted the odd hours, the difficult calls, and the quiet heaviness that comes home from circuit work, thank you for being my own continuity.

Table of Contents

Preface: Why This Book, Why Now

This book began as a series of notes written in hotel rooms, late at night, after court had adjourned and the day's interviews had ended, when the only sound was the heater cycling and the wind pressing lightly against the window. I wrote to remember details that would otherwise blur: the rhythm of circuit days, the small acts of dignity that held fragile situations together, and the quiet ways that distance reshaped everything the justice and health systems tried to do.

At first, I assumed the notes were only for me. Circuit work is intense and transient. You arrive, you assess, you testify, you write, you leave. The plane always leaves. The cases continue without you. It felt important to capture what I was seeing, not as a record of individual lives, but as a record of patterns: how risk is amplified by geography, how "reasonable" conditions become impossible in small places, how remand can function as a holding pattern created by weather and scarcity, and how the hotel can become an improvised clinical unit when there is nowhere else for the work to go.

Over time, I realized the notes were also answering a larger question: What does justice look like when roads disappear? Not justice as a slogan, but justice as lived experience by victims, accused persons, families, and the local professionals who hold the system together with unsung labor. The Arctic exposes the gap between what systems promise and what they can deliver. It does so without malice and without apology. Distance makes everything honest.

Why now? Because the pressures that shaped the stories in these pages are not fading. Housing shortages, staff turnover, substance-related harms, trauma exposure, and gaps in mental health and addiction services remain persistent realities across many northern communities. Meanwhile, courts continue to require clear answers about fitness, risk, responsibility, and sentencing, often on compressed timelines, with limited collateral, and in settings where interpretation and culturally safe practice are essential. The result is a recurring ethical tension: the system asks for certainty and continuity, while geography supplies neither.

I am writing this book for several audiences at once.

For clinicians and trainees, it is a portrait of forensic practice in a setting that refuses shortcuts, where cultural safety is not a slogan, where confidentiality is a daily discipline, and where recommendations must survive real constraints or risk becoming traps.

For justice professionals, it is a ground-level view of how conditions, remand, and diversion function differently when anonymity is impossible and services are intermittent, along with what tends to work better when the goal is genuine safety rather than predictable breach cycles.

For policymakers and administrators, it is a reminder that continuity is not a luxury in the North; it is the intervention, and that capacity-building models matter more than occasional specialist visits.

And for general readers, it is a human account of a system that is both intimate and strained: people doing their best, often with too few options, in a place where the weather can overrule the best plans.

This is not a book of heroic medicine. It is a book about limits—clinical limits, system limits, and personal limits—and about the quiet responsibility of trying to do good work inside those limits without pretending they don't exist. It is also a book about respect: for the communities who live in the North year-round and for the local staff whose steadiness is the true infrastructure of care.

Because these stories are drawn from real patterns, the vignettes are written as composites. Names, timelines, charges, and identifying details have been altered or blended to protect privacy and prevent re-identification. The aim is not to expose individuals. The aim is to illuminate the intersection where law, mental health, and geography meet, and to ask how we can build systems that are more realistic, more humane, and more effective.

Why this book? Because the Arctic taught me that distance is not a backdrop. It is an active force in justice and care.

Why now? Because we cannot keep pretending that southern templates automatically fit northern realities, and because better is possible when we design for the place we are actually in.

The plane will always leave.

The question is what we leave behind.

Note on Language, Place Names, and Permissions

This book is written with care for the realities of small northern communities, where anonymity is limited and words travel quickly. Because the stories in these pages draw from real patterns of practice, I have taken deliberate steps to protect privacy and avoid unintended harm.

Language and Tone

I use person-first language wherever possible (e.g., "a person in custody," "a person living with psychosis," "a person with substance use disorder"), while recognizing that some readers and communities may prefer identity-first language in certain contexts. When legal terms are necessary (e.g., accused, complainant, remand, fitness, NCRMD), they are used for clarity and consistency with court processes, not to reduce anyone to a label.

I also distinguish between cultural practices and clinical symptoms. Spiritual beliefs, traditional healing, silence, indirect communication, and community-specific ways of expressing distress are not treated as pathology. Where uncertainty exists, I name it explicitly rather than assuming a "southern" interpretation is correct.

Place Names and Community Identifiers

To reduce the risk of re-identification, many place names have been generalized, blended, or used sparingly, especially in vignettes that involve unusual events, high-profile matters, or distinctive personal details. In some sections, I refer to "the community," "the regional center," or "the circuit" rather than naming a specific location. Where a real location is named (for example, as part of my own travel narrative), it is presented in a way that avoids linking identifiable individuals to specific cases.

Vignettes As Composites

All clinical and legal vignettes are composites. Identifying details, including names, ages, family structures, occupations, timelines, charges, and outcomes, have been altered, merged, or omitted. No vignette is intended to represent a single individual or a single case. The purpose is to convey recurring themes and ethical tensions in northern forensic work, not to document any person's story.

Permissions and Acknowledgments

Individuals and organizations are acknowledged by name only with explicit permission. In settings where naming could risk identification or cause unintended consequences, acknowledgments are expressed in general terms (e.g., "court workers," "nursing staff," "interpreters," "community wellness teams"). Any quotations attributed to individuals are paraphrased, composite, or included only with permission.

Ethical Intent

The intent of these safeguards is simple: to respect the dignity and privacy of the people and communities whose realities shaped this work, while still speaking honestly about the system-level challenges and the practical solutions that determine whether justice and care can truly hold in the Arctic.

If this book has errors of emphasis, I hope they are errors of humility rather than certainty.

Glossary

Accused - The person charged with an offense (the term used in Canadian criminal proceedings).

Adjournment - A court appearance or hearing postponed to a later date.

Aftercare - Follow-up supports after discharge from hospital or release from custody.

Bail - Release from custody while awaiting trial or sentencing, usually with conditions.

Bail plan - A practical plan describing where the person will live, who will support them, and how risks will be managed while on release.

Breach - Failure to comply with a court order or release condition (may result in new charges or return to custody).

Capacity - The ability to understand relevant information and appreciate reasonably foreseeable consequences; capacity is decision-specific and may fluctuate.

Collateral information - Information from sources other than the person being assessed (e.g., records, family, police reports, prior assessments).

Conditions - Court-ordered rules (e.g., curfew, no-contact, abstinence, reporting); conditions may reduce harm or create predictable failure if unrealistic.

Confidentiality - The duty to protect private information; in forensic contexts, confidentiality is limited by the legal purpose of the assessment and how the report may be used.

Coercive control - A pattern of domination in an intimate relationship using intimidation, isolation, threats, surveillance, and control of resources (with or without physical violence).

Composite vignette - A narrative blended from multiple real-world patterns, with identifying details altered or omitted to prevent re-identification.

Court coordinator - Staff who manage scheduling, logistics, and the flow of court matters (titles vary by jurisdiction).

Court worker - A community-based support person who helps individuals navigate court processes, understand orders, and connect with services; often a key bridge in northern systems.

Crisis stabilization - Short-term interventions aimed at restoring safety and basic functioning (e.g., sleep, withdrawal support, de-escalation, medication continuity).

De-escalation - Strategies to reduce agitation and prevent conflict or violence (pacing, tone, space, choices, calming routines, safe exits).

Delirium - An acute, fluctuating disturbance in attention and cognition, usually due to a medical cause or intoxication/withdrawal; a medical emergency.

Disposition - A legal outcome or decision about what happens next (e.g., sentence, release, or a Review Board disposition under mental disorder provisions).

Diversion - Redirecting a person from deeper justice involvement toward treatment or support when appropriate, with safeguards and monitoring.

Dual relationship - When a professional relationship overlaps with another relationship (social, family, community), creating boundary and confidentiality complexity.

Dynamic risk factors - Changeable factors linked to risk (e.g., intoxication, acute psychosis, unstable housing, conflict, insomnia).

Executive function - Brain-based skills that support planning, impulse control, working memory, task completion, and self-monitoring.

Expert witness - A clinician qualified to provide opinion evidence to the court within their scope of expertise.

Fitness to stand trial - Whether an accused can understand the nature and object of the proceedings and communicate meaningfully with counsel (legal thresholds are jurisdiction-specific).

Formulation - A structured clinical explanation of how symptoms, history, and context fit together to inform risk and care planning.

Harm reduction - Approaches that reduce injury and death even when substance use continues (e.g., relapse planning, safer-use supports, non-punitive re-engagement).

Hamlet - A small northern community; in Nunavut, also a formal municipal designation.

Interpreter - A person who translates spoken language during interviews, court, or care; interpretation quality and conflicts of interest can affect accuracy.

Intoxication - Acute effects of substance use that may impair memory, judgment, and behavior; relevant to reliability and risk.

Land-based supports - Community-led cultural and wellness activities rooted in land, language, and traditional practices (where available and defined by the community).

Least restrictive alternative - A principle of choosing the option that protects safety while limiting liberty as little as reasonably possible.

Medevac / evacuation - Medical transport (often by air) to a larger center for assessment or treatment not available locally; may reduce acute harm while creating relational and cultural disruption.

Mental disorder provisions - Canadian criminal law framework governing fitness assessments, NCRMD findings, and Review Board dispositions (Criminal Code, Part XX.1).

Moral injury - Distress that arises when one cannot carry out what one believes is right due to system constraints (scarcity, geography, capacity limits).

No-contact order - A condition prohibiting contact with a named person; in small communities, "no contact" may be difficult to operationalize without realistic avoidance strategies.

NCRMD (Not Criminally Responsible on account of Mental Disorder) - A legal finding that a person is not criminally responsible due to mental disorder at the time of the offense; the person is typically managed under Review Board oversight rather than a standard conviction or sentence.

Probation - Community supervision following sentence, with conditions and monitoring.

Protective factors - Factors that reduce the likelihood of harm (e.g., stable housing, supportive relationships, treatment engagement, structured routine).

Remand - Custody while awaiting trial or sentencing (not a sentence); in remote settings, remand may be prolonged by geography, service gaps, and weather.

Review Board - A specialized tribunal that makes decisions for people found NCRMD or unfit, focusing on public safety, liberty, and treatment needs.

Risk assessment - Evaluation of the likelihood and severity of future harm (e.g., violence, self-harm, relapse, victimization), considering both person-level and context-level variables.

Safety plan - A stepwise plan to reduce risk (warning signs, coping steps, supports, emergency contacts, crisis options).

Sally port - A secure, controlled entry area in a jail where movement in and out is managed for safety.

Segregation - Isolation from the general custody population; may be used for safety but can worsen mental health and cognition.

Sentencing report - A report informing the court about mental health, risk, and rehabilitative needs relevant to sentencing (formats vary).

Shared care - A model in which multiple providers or teams coordinate care (e.g., local services + remote specialist + justice supports) with defined roles and continuity.

Static risk factors - Historical, unchangeable factors (e.g., past violence) that inform baseline risk but do not explain day-to-day fluctuations.

Structured professional judgment (SPJ) - An approach that combines evidence-based risk factors with transparent clinical reasoning and scenario-based planning.

Tele-forensics - Forensic assessment or consultation delivered remotely (video or phone), ideally paired with strong local anchoring and clear follow-up ownership.

Therapeutic jurisprudence - A legal approach that considers the therapeutic or harmful effects of legal processes and aims to support rehabilitation while maintaining justice and safety.

Trauma-informed practice - Care that prioritizes safety, trust, choice, collaboration, and empowerment, while recognizing trauma's impact without excusing harmful behavior.

Treatment order - A court-linked directive requiring engagement with treatment (varies by jurisdiction and legal authority).

Vicarious trauma - The impact on helpers exposed to others' trauma, often accumulating over time in small systems with repeated crises.

Victim services - Supports for victims or complainants (e.g., safety planning, court navigation, counseling referrals, information).

Warm handover - A direct, relational transfer of care (introducing the person to the next provider or support), rather than relying on the person to navigate a referral alone.

Acronyms and Abbreviations

NCRMD - Not Criminally Responsible on account of Mental Disorder

SPJ - Structured Professional Judgment

PART I

ARRIVAL: LEARNING THE NORTH

CHAPTER 1

The Flight North

Winter 2010.

Ottawa was still asleep when I arrived at the airport, the kind of early darkness that feels permanent until you remember it is only temporary, only winter, only this hour. Inside the terminal, the light was fluorescent and steady, too clean, too certain. People moved with the practiced speed of travelers who knew where they were going. I did too, technically. I had a ticket with my name on it and a destination printed in bold: Iqaluit.

But knowing the destination is not the same as knowing what the destination will ask of you.

At the gate, I watched the faces around me, some seasoned, some tired, some quietly excited. There were parkas folded over arms, duffel bags that looked practical rather than stylish, boots with salt stains. A few conversations carried the soft shorthand of people returning to a place they already belonged, quick updates, shared names, plans that assumed continuity. I sat with my file folder and my thoughts, aware of how little continuity I could claim.

I was going north for the first time as a visiting forensic psychiatrist. The words sounded official in the way credentials often do, and yet I felt the opposite of official. I felt provisional. Borrowed. Like someone holding a tool they understood in theory but had never used in this particular climate.

The boarding announcement came, and the line formed with quiet efficiency. There are flights where the plane is simply a vehicle. This did not feel like one of those. This felt like a crossing.

Three hours from Ottawa to Iqaluit, three hours on paper, three hours in a world where minutes can stretch and compress depending on what they carry. I stepped onto the aircraft and paused, surprised by the layout. The cabin was divided in a way I had not experienced before, with a clear separation between cargo and passenger sections. The partition was not just a structural feature; it felt symbolic, a reminder that this route served multiple realities at once. People and supplies. Necessities and narratives. The north does not receive luxury first; it receives what keeps life moving.

I found my seat and settled in. The hum of preparation, the shifting of bags, the brief, polite negotiations for overhead space, familiar rituals. But beyond them, a different awareness began to form, that this flight was part of an ecosystem. An artery.

As we lifted off, Ottawa fell away with a softness that almost looked like peace. Then the landscape changed. The world below became a study in white and distance, snow, ice, and the stark geometry of frozen waterways. The longer we flew, the more the earth seemed to simplify itself, stripping away the distractions of roads and dense neighborhoods and the comforting evidence of proximity.

Up here, there was nowhere to hide, not for the land, and eventually, not for the work.

The first impressions were physical before they were philosophical: sky, ice, distance.

The sky was enormous in a way southern skies rarely are. It did not just hang over the world; it held it. The light had that winter clarity that makes everything sharper, less forgiving. Below, ice spread like a language written across the terrain, cracked in some places, smooth in others, layered in subtle tones you do not notice until you are forced to stare long enough to see the difference between white and white and white.

And the distance, distance was not a measurement here. It was a condition.

Somewhere in that suspended space, as the plane steadied and the cabin settled into its mid-flight rhythm, the air hostesses began service. It startled me, not because service is unusual on a flight, but because it was so good, so attentive, so complete. They moved through the aisle with practiced grace, offering a full-course meal, not a token sandwich in plastic, but something complex enough to feel like an assertion: you will be cared for on this route. It was not indulgence. It was sustenance.

There was also coffee, special coffee, the kind that arrives with options, not assumptions. And then, later, warm cookies, soft in the middle, the scent drifting briefly through the cabin like a small domestic miracle. In that moment, high above the white landscape, the warmth of a cookie felt oddly significant. It was comfort delivered with intention. It said: this journey matters enough for us to do this well.

I watched the crew and felt a quiet respect. They were not visitors. They belonged to this corridor between worlds, navigating it repeatedly, making it humane through small acts done consistently. Their competence was casual, almost invisible, and that invisibility felt like a lesson: in the north, the most essential work is often the least dramatic.

I ate slowly, half from appetite, half from trying to anchor myself in something tangible. Somewhere beneath the routine of cutlery and cups, my mind kept returning to the word *visitor*.

Visiting.

It sounds gentle, almost social. Like a trip made for pleasure. But in forensic psychiatry, "visiting" carries a different weight. It means you arrive with authority that is partly borrowed, borrowed from law, from institutions, from the expectations of systems that want answers. You arrive to assess people whose lives may be hanging in the balance of language: fitness, responsibility, risk, capacity, mitigation. Words that can alter the shape of someone's future.

And you arrive knowing you will leave.

That is the uneasy truth at the center of the visitor identity. In the south, you can pretend continuity will appear if you just try hard enough. In the Arctic, the limits are visible immediately. Flights are scheduled around weather. Clinics are scheduled around staffing. Courts are scheduled around circuits. Everything is timed to scarcity.

I stared out the window and let the discomfort sit where it belonged. There is a kind of arrogance that can come disguised as professionalism, a belief that competence alone is enough to justify presence. I did not want that disguise. I wanted to arrive with the only posture that seemed remotely honest: humility, uncertainty, and purpose, in that order.

Humility, because I was stepping into a place with histories I did not own and harms I did not fully understand.

Uncertainty, because forensic work thrives on questions that do not resolve neatly, and the north adds layers of context that a textbook cannot anticipate.

Purpose, because despite everything, I was not going north to admire the scenery. I was going because people needed assessment and care, and because systems, imperfect as they were, still required someone to do the work with care and rigor.

The pilot announced our descent, and the cabin shifted again. People sat up straighter. Jackets came out. Conversations paused. The plane angled downward, and the landscape rose to meet us.

Iqaluit appeared not as a sprawling metropolis but as a presence, structures gathered against the vastness, a community placed with intention in a world that does not make things easy. We touched down, and the wheels made a sound that felt like punctuation.

When the door opened, the cold entered like a fact.

Not the cold of Ottawa that bites and then relents, but a cold that seemed to have its own intelligence, dry, sharp, unnegotiable. It moved into lungs and made every breath feel deliberate. The air smelled clean, almost metallic. I stood at the threshold for a moment longer than necessary, letting my body register that this was not a colder version of home. This was a different environment altogether.

It was about 1 p.m. when I arrived, the light already beginning its slow winter drift toward early evening. The sky had that pale clarity that makes time hard to read. I collected my things and followed the flow of passengers into the small, efficient terminal.

Outside, taxis waited with the practical patience of people used to weather. I shared a taxi with another traveler, someone who seemed to know the rhythm here, the unspoken rules. Bags were placed without fuss, doors shut with a solid finality, and we pulled away from the airport into the wide, crisp day.

The ride to the Frobisher Hotel was short but memorable. The landscape passed in clean lines, snow-packed ground, buildings set against the open space, the sense that everything here had been earned rather than assumed. The roads felt purposeful. The town felt real, not romantic. It did not perform itself for visitors.

As we approached the hotel, I felt that familiar professional tightening in my chest, the quiet awareness that once you check in, you are no longer simply a traveler. You are a person with responsibilities waiting behind the next door, the next phone call, the next list of names.

The taxi stopped. The driver helped with the luggage in a way that was efficient but not rushed. I stepped out and looked up at the building, ordinary in shape, extraordinary in what it represented for me in that moment. A base. A temporary anchor. A place where I would sleep, write, think, and prepare to enter courtrooms and correctional spaces where the stakes are never theoretical.

Inside, warmth wrapped around me. The lobby held the soft noise of life, people arriving, leaving, waiting. I signed in, took my key, and stood for a moment longer than necessary, letting myself feel the strangeness of it.

Hotel rooms usually represent anonymity. Here, I suspected anonymity would be a luxury I would not have.

As I walked toward the elevator, I felt the "visitor" identity settle more firmly on my shoulders, not as a burden, exactly, but as a responsibility that required constant attention. I would need to watch my assumptions. Watch my pace. Watch my language. I would need to respect the fact that I was entering a place where relationships mattered more than credentials, where people remembered how you behaved long after they forgot what you said.

Upstairs, in the quiet of my room, I set my bag down and looked out the window. The world outside was bright and cold and vast. Somewhere beyond the hotel walls were the court, the jail, the community, the files, and the lives behind them.

I took off my coat slowly, as if the act itself might help me transition from traveler to clinician, from passenger to witness.

There is a moment at the beginning of certain journeys when you realize you cannot be the same person on the other side. You might try, but the place will not allow it. The Arctic, its sky, its ice, its distance, does not merely host you. It changes the terms of who you are.

And so I stood there, on my first winter trip north in 2010, in a hotel room in Iqaluit, and accepted what I could not yet fully name:

I had arrived as a visitor.

Now I would have to earn whatever right I had to do the work.

CHAPTER 2

Clinic Without Walls

I arrived on a Sunday, the kind of day that is supposed to be quiet, an unofficial pause before the machinery of the week begins. In the south, Sunday has a predictable shape: errands, rest, maybe a little dread about Monday. In the Arctic, Sunday had a different logic. It was not a day off. It was a day of positioning, a day when the work began without formally announcing itself.

Not long after I checked into the hotel, the court staff arrived.

They came to the lobby with the calm efficiency of people who had done this many times before, carrying what I had come for: depositions, documents, the paper trail of other people's lives. The stack was not dramatic, but it was heavy in the way paper can be heavy when it carries consequences. We exchanged greetings, brief and professional, and then the files were in my hands and the staff were gone, back into their world of schedules, logistics, and public-facing order.

I returned to my room with that familiar sense of being a temporary node in a larger system. A visiting forensic psychiatrist. A name on a circuit. A person brought in to interpret, to clarify, to assess, sometimes to give the system what it believes it needs: an opinion.

I laid the depositions out on the small desk by the window like someone preparing a map. I read slowly, making notes, underlining phrases that seemed ordinary but might carry hidden meaning in court. Dates. Prior charges. Brief descriptions of events. Repeated references to alcohol, to arguments, to "uncooperative behavior." Words that appear so frequently in the criminal file that they can begin to feel like placeholders.

But placeholders are dangerous. They flatten people.

And I had come north to do the opposite, to take the flatness of a file and search, as carefully as possible, for the contours of a human being.

Outside, the light faded quickly. Winter darkness does not drift; it arrives. It moves in with a kind of certainty that feels almost administrative. One moment the town is lit with pale daytime clarity; the next it is swallowed in shadow and streetlights and the dim glow of windows. In the south, darkness can feel like atmosphere. Here, it felt like infrastructure, something you plan around, something you respect.

By the time I looked up from my notes, the day had already folded itself into night.

I went down to the hotel restaurant for dinner, needing something warm and simple to interrupt the tunnel of reading. The dining room had that familiar hotel quiet: soft voices, clink of cutlery, the muted hum of a television somewhere. People ate without lingering, as if the night outside encouraged efficiency. I ordered, ate, and I was out. The rhythm of this place was already teaching me: do what you need to do, do not waste energy, move with purpose.

On the way back, I saw them.

A couple standing outside in the brutal cold, minus 54 degrees Celsius, smoking.

They were not rushing. They were not performing toughness. They were simply there, hands tucked in, shoulders slightly hunched, exhaling smoke into air so cold it seemed to crystallize the breath itself. I slowed down without meaning to. The sight was jarring, not because I had not seen people smoke in winter before, but because this cold was not ordinary winter. This was the kind of cold that makes you understand why humans invented shelter, why survival is not a metaphor here.

And yet there they were, exposed, because nicotine does not negotiate.

It hit me with unexpected force: the power-hold of addiction.

Not as an abstract concept, not as a diagnostic checkbox, not as a line in a chart, nicotine dependence. But as a lived demand strong enough to pull people out of warmth and into danger, strong enough to make a person stand in a temperature that can injure skin in minutes, simply to satisfy an urge that the body insists is necessary.

I went back inside carrying that image like a clinical lesson with no lecture attached.

This was the clinic without walls.

In the south, "access" can mean wait times, referral pathways, clinic capacity, insurance coverage. Here, access meant something more elemental. It meant whether a plane could land. Whether a road was passable, if a road even existed. Whether the nurse was on shift. Whether the phone line worked. Whether the person you needed to see was in town, or had been transferred, or had simply disappeared into the weather and the distances that swallow plans.

In the Arctic, you do not just schedule care. You negotiate it, daily, hourly, against forces that do not care about your calendar.

Weather is not a background condition. It is an active participant.

Planes are not a convenience. They are a lifeline.

Phones are not supplemental. They are sometimes the only bridge.

And shortages are not occasional disruptions; they are part of the operating system.

That night, back in my room, I returned to the depositions with a different awareness. It was not just the cases. It was the context that would shape every interview and every conclusion I might be asked to draw.

If someone missed appointments, was it "noncompliance," or was it a storm, a cancelled flight, a broken phone, a caregiver overwhelmed, a lack of money, a lack of transportation, a lack of privacy?

If someone breached conditions, was it "defiance," or was it a condition that made no sense in a place where everyone is connected, where housing is crowded, where the very architecture of life makes separation impossible?

If someone was intoxicated, was it "poor choices," or was it also grief, trauma, boredom, pain, a lack of treatment options, a lack of alternatives?

The more I read, the more the files began to sound less like individual stories and more like echoes of a system trying to function at the edge of geography.

I wrote notes late into the evening. Not because I wanted to be thorough, though I did, but because the night had already taught me something important: when you are visiting, you have less time than you think, and the conditions can change without warning.

The rhythm of care here was not Monday to Friday.

It was weather to weather.

It was flight to flight.

It was connection to disconnection.

It was the availability of a human being who might be the only nurse on duty, the only interpreter available, the only officer who knew how to calm a person down, the only counsellor who could keep someone from unraveling.

It was a rhythm shaped by scarcity and sustained by people who kept showing up anyway.

At some point, I put down my pen and looked out at the darkness beyond the window. The town lights were small points against a vast blackness. Somewhere out there were the people whose names filled my notes. Somewhere out there were the courtrooms and holding cells and families waiting. Somewhere out there were smokers in −54 °C, because addiction is indifferent to comfort and indifferent to consequence.

And I realized that "clinic" was too small a word for what I was stepping into.

This was care stretched across distance.

This was justice moving on circuits.

This was psychiatry practiced with interruptions built in.

A clinic without walls, because walls require stability, and stability is not always available here.

I turned back to the files, more careful now with every assumption, and more aware of what I would need to carry into the week: not just clinical knowledge, but humility about the logistics of survival.

In places like this, access is not a policy slogan.

It is the difference between help that arrives, and help that never does.

CHAPTER 3

First Calls: Court, Jail, Nursing Station

Monday morning arrived with the quiet decisiveness of a place that does not wait for you to feel ready.

Downstairs, the hotel breakfast room was already in motion, people moving with purpose, boots drying near the entrance, coats draped over chairs as if no one expected to linger. I fixed a plate: Eggs Benedict, a small luxury that felt almost theatrical against the hard geometry of the Arctic outside. There was coffee, strong and necessary. And there was fresh fruit that was anything but fresh, soft around the edges, tired in color, flown-in optimism that had lost its argument somewhere between warehouses and weather delays.

It was a small, ordinary reminder of how "normal" arrives here: late, expensive, imperfect, and still appreciated.

I drank my coffee and watched the room. There is a particular kind of concentration on Monday mornings in remote settings, the sense that whatever can be done today must be done today, because tomorrow might be cancelled by wind, darkness, or a plane that does not come. People here learn early not to gamble on continuity.

Back upstairs, I made the first call that mattered.

A quick telephone call to the jail to announce my intention to visit at 10 a.m., and to confirm that I would be coming with an interpreter. It was not the kind of call you make in the south, where access is assumed and schedules are firm. Here, even a simple visit required coordination: staff availability, escort availability, room availability, interpreter availability. A visit was not just a clinical decision; it was logistics.

The person on the other end was courteous, concise. There was no unnecessary conversation. We both knew what the call meant: a visitor was coming into custody space, and the institution would make room, if it could.

I hung up and glanced at my notes. The day's work had three anchors, three destinations that would shape everything I did and everything I could not do.

Court.

Jail.

Nursing station.

Justice, custody, care.

It sounds clean when you put it into a triad. It sounds almost structured, almost manageable. But in practice, the triad is not three separate lanes. It is one narrow road with traffic coming from both directions. Court wants clarity. Jail wants safety. Nursing stations want continuity. And the people at the center of it all want, often, desperately, relief.

Sometimes they also want vindication. Or freedom. Or to be left alone. Or to be heard for the first time.

And then there is the visitor, me, trying to navigate all of it with limited time, borrowed authority, and the awareness that every conclusion I write might become a lever in someone else's hands.

By midmorning, I was outside, waiting for a taxi.

It arrived already carrying multiple passengers. In Iqaluit, taxis do not always belong to one person at a time. They belong to the day, to the movement of a small community where efficiency is part of survival. I climbed in, shifting my bag of notes, nodding greetings to strangers whose faces I would likely see again, at the store, in the lobby, perhaps even in court. In small places, you learn quickly that "private life" is not a stable category.

As the taxi pulled away, something unexpected happened. The motion, the closeness of shared transport, the rhythm of passing streets, something about it unlocked a memory so vivid it felt like stepping into another life.

I thought of taxi rides between Lantoro and Aro.

Long before I was a visiting forensic psychiatrist in the Arctic, I had been a psychiatric resident travelling those routes in Nigeria, back and forth, learning my craft in places that were also shaped by scarcity, but a different kind of scarcity. I remembered the feel of those rides: the way roads carry stories, the way a vehicle becomes a moving confessional, the way time stretches when you are on your way to something you do not fully understand yet.

I remembered being at the World Health Organization training center in Aro, Abeokuta, the intensity of learning, the early confidence of youth mixed with the quiet terror of responsibility. I remembered how training changes you, not by giving you certainty, but by teaching you how to work in uncertainty without lying to yourself.

And then, as if the mind insists on mapping its migrations, my thoughts leapt forward.

Merseyside. Warrington, Leighton, Maghull, Liverpool. Residency again, this time as a Royal College of Psychiatrists overseas doctor, stepping into a system that looked familiar on paper but moved to a different tempo in practice. The same human distress, the same need for containment and care, but new ward cultures, new multidisciplinary rituals, new risk language, new thresholds for admission and discharge, and documentation that demanded a different kind of precision. I learned quickly that competence had to be demonstrated twice: first in the clinic, and again in the grammar of the system.

The change was not only clinical; it was cultural. Accents reshaped familiar words. Expectations often lived between lines, how to speak in handover and ward rounds, how to frame uncertainty, what counted as "enough" history, what a supervisor meant by "keep an eye," how disagreement could be expressed without sounding combative. It was work, yes, but it was also translation, learning what travelled well from home training, and what needed to be rebuilt to fit the UK's rhythms of psychiatry and the Royal College's standards.

Immigration, in that sense, became a second kind of residency: learning new systems, new accents, new expectations. Finding your footing again. Learning which parts of you translate easily and which parts require reinvention.

And then, finally:

Canada.

The country where I would become, eventually, someone who flew north on circuit trips, carrying files, making assessments, writing opinions with consequences.

In the taxi, layered in winter clothing, heading toward the jail in Iqaluit, I felt those geographies overlap for a moment: Nigeria, the UK, Canada. Roads and flights. Places where institutions try to contain suffering. Places where clinicians try to relieve it. Places where human beings keep being human no matter what system surrounds them.

The taxi slowed at an intersection. The driver took a turn without hesitation. I pulled my thoughts back to the present.

Because this was the reality of the Monday ahead: the triad of the trip did not allow for much drifting.

Court would demand precision. Timelines. Diagnoses. Capacities. Risks.

Jail would demand practicality. Safety rules. Limited time. Limited space. Limited privacy.

The nursing station would demand collaboration. Assessment. Medication continuity. Crisis planning.

And I would have to negotiate not only my schedule, but my presence, where I was allowed to stand, how long I was allowed to speak, what I was allowed to ask, what could be safely documented, and how quickly an interpretation could be trusted when words do not translate neatly across languages and worlds.

Even space was not neutral here.

An interview room is not just a room. It is a controlled environment, a balance of risk and dignity. A hallway is not just a hallway. It is a place where confidentiality can dissolve with a single passing face. A nursing station is not just a nursing station. It is sometimes a single overworked nurse with a phone and a list of people who need help.

Time, too, had a different character.

In visiting work, time is always scarce. In the Arctic, time is fragile. Weather can erase your plans. Delays can multiply. The person you came to see might be transferred, asleep, intoxicated, too distressed, or simply unavailable because the system is stretched thin.

You learn to treat every completed assessment as a small victory against entropy.

The taxi came to a stop. The jail was ahead, solid, functional, unimpressed by my reflections. I paid my share, stepped out into the cold, and adjusted my gloves.

I checked my watch.

It was not yet 10, but I could feel the day already tightening into its narrow corridor of tasks.

Court.

Jail.

Nursing station.

Justice.

Custody.

Care.

I walked toward the entrance, carrying my notes, carrying my history, carrying the strange privilege and burden of being the visitor who arrives, asks questions, writes conclusions, and then, eventually, leaves.

CHAPTER 4

Introductions and Protocol

In places built on distance, introductions are not a formality. They are a method.

On my first Monday, I learned quickly that the Arctic does not run on job titles alone. It runs on people, people who know where the keys are, who know who is in custody, who is likely to be in court, who is grieving, who is safe to approach first, and what cannot be done on a particular day because weather or staffing has already decided otherwise.

The formal itinerary might say court, jail, nursing station, but the real map is human. And the first rule of visiting forensic work in the North is this: you do not arrive as the center of the system. You arrive as a guest inside it.

That is where Ms. J comes in.

Let's call the court coordinator Ms. J. She was younger than I expected, energetic, composed, and unmistakably hardworking, the kind of person whose competence is not loud but constant. She had made the North a home, not a posting. A place to raise her daughters. A place where her dogs mattered as much as her job. And that detail, dogs, was not incidental. In the Arctic, the presence of dogs tells you something about how a person has decided to live.

There are places where dogs are pets.

And then there are places where dogs are part of the landscape, companions, protectors, working animals, symbols of endurance, reminders that life here has always been negotiated with cold, movement, and the need for warmth that is not only physical. Even when a dog is simply a family dog, the relationship feels different in an environment where the outdoors can punish carelessness. Dogs in the Arctic are not just loved; they are respected.

Ms. J spoke about her daughters and her dogs in the same tone she used for court schedules and logistics, matter-of-fact, committed, practical. That, too, felt like a northern style of love: not sentimental, but steady.

Ms. J became my first true point of orientation. Not because she was in charge of me, she wasn't, but because she knew how the pieces fit together, and she understood that visiting professionals often arrive with an internal script that does not match local reality.

She also did something small that mattered enormously: she made movement possible.

She drove me back and forth in a Dodge truck, from court to the hotel and back again, navigating the town with the ease of someone who had learned its rhythm in every season. The truck itself felt like a northern argument: built for function, not appearance. Sturdy. Unapologetic. Capable of carrying what needed to be carried.

In the south, a ride might be just a ride. Here, it was part of protocol.

In the back and forth, I learned the unspoken rules: where to enter, where to wait, who needed to be notified, what time meant in a system shaped by delays, and how to avoid becoming an inconvenience in a place where everyone was already doing the work of three people. Ms. J did not lecture. She simply modelled the reality.

This was how introductions happened, not through speeches, but through logistics.

At court, she introduced me to a network that would become essential:

- Guards, whose job was safety and whose judgment could determine whether an interview was possible that day.
- Court workers, who understood the community context, the family lines, the unstated histories that never make it into affidavits.
- Interpreters, who carried more than language, who carried meaning, nuance, and the ethical weight of translating a person's inner life into words that the court could understand.
- Victim services, whose presence reminded me that every forensic file is not only about the accused. It is also about harm, fear, survival, and the long echo of an event in someone else's life.
- Nurses, often the quiet backbone of the entire system, bridging care and custody and community with whatever tools they had on hand.

It would have been easy to treat these introductions as procedural, names, roles, handshakes. But I sensed early that the protocol here was not just about access.

It was about respect.

Respect for the people who stay.

Respect for the people whose lives are being assessed.

Respect for the limits of time, of space, of privacy, of resources.

And respect for knowledge, especially the knowledge that does not appear in textbooks.

One of the most important lessons Ms. J taught me, without ever stating it outright, was this: in the Arctic, knowledge is distributed. It does not sit in one office, one chart, or one credentialed person. It lives in the relationships between staff, in the memory of the nurse who remembers who decompensates in the dark, in the court worker who knows which family is in crisis, in the interpreter who knows which words cannot be said directly without shame.

If you want to do forensic work responsibly here, you have to learn who holds what knowledge, and how to ask for it respectfully.

Not every question is yours to ask immediately.

Not every answer belongs in your notes.

And not every insight is something you are entitled to extract simply because you have been invited north.

Ms. J was also, in her own way, part of what made the Arctic feel survivable for me. Her humor, dry and practical, cut through my internal seriousness. Her hospitality, quiet and functional, made the trip feel less like an extraction and more like a collaboration.

Over time, I began to understand something else: hospitality in the North is not always expressed as warmth in words. It is expressed as help.

A ride when you need one.

An introduction that clears the path.

A reminder not to schedule something during a time when the interpreter is already booked.

A "just so you know" comment that prevents a mistake.

Ms. J's presence, and the way she handled the impossible details of circuit days, did something subtle to my nervous system. It made the Arctic less intimidating. Less foreign. It made it feel, if not like home, then like a place where I could return and do good work without being swallowed by the logistics.

And I did return.

For the next decade and a half, I came back again and again, long after that first winter trip had faded into a set of stored impressions: sky, ice, distance, and a hotel desk covered in depositions.

Even after Ms. J eventually left, the memory of her made something in the Arctic remain warm for me. Not in a sentimental way, but in a professional one: the warmth of being treated as a human being while doing work that is often heavy and impersonal. The warmth of a system that, despite its constraints, still finds ways to welcome the visitor, so long as the visitor remembers to be humble.

That was the real protocol.

Not simply where to stand in court, or how to schedule a jail visit.

But how to enter a place with respect, to learn its rhythm, and to remember, always, that the people who live and work here are not supporting characters in your story.

They are the story.

And you are only passing through.

PART II

PEOPLE, PLACE, AND THE CLINICAL REALITY

CHAPTER 5

Circuit Court Days

Circuit court days begin before court begins.

They start in the hotel lobby, in the thin hours when people move quietly, coats pulled tight, eyes already scanning for who is present and who is missing. They start in taxis that pick up more than one passenger at a time, and in hallways where the same small cluster of professionals—court staff, counsel, escorts, interpreters—reassemble like a travelling theatre troupe. The difference is that what is staged here is not entertainment. It is consequence.

By the time you walk into the courthouse, the day already has momentum.

The courtroom has its own rhythm, and on circuit that rhythm is both familiar and precarious. There is a docket. There are names. There are matters that look simple on paper and prove complicated in a sentence. And there is an unspoken pressure hovering over everything: we have to get through what we can today, because tomorrow might not belong to us.

A flight could be cancelled. Weather could ground the circuit. A witness might not arrive. An accused person might be transferred. An interpreter might be pulled into an emergency elsewhere. In the Arctic, the court calendar is always written in pencil, no matter how official it appears.

The morning begins with what looks, to an outsider, like routine: calling matters, confirming appearances, setting dates. But the routine is constantly interrupted by the North.

A matter is adjourned because counsel is stuck somewhere between communities, grounded by wind.

Another is delayed because disclosure has not arrived, because mail, planes, and the slow logistics of distance are not excuses here; they are facts.

Someone does not appear because transportation did not happen, because someone forgot, because someone could not get out of bed, because someone is intoxicated, because someone is unwell, because someone is afraid.

Court in the Arctic is not less serious than court in the south. In some ways, it is more serious because the margin for error is thinner. When you only have court in town at certain intervals, delay is not measured in days. It is measured in seasons.

You can feel that pressure in the room.

It sits behind the judge's patience, behind the lawyers' urgency, behind the quiet efficiency of the court coordinator, behind the steady presence of sheriffs and guards. Everyone understands that time is limited and the docket is long. The system, already stretched, becomes even tighter on circuit days.

And yet, for all its urgency, the courtroom is also intimate.

In large southern courts, anonymity is built into the architecture. People are one case among many, one face in a crowd that constantly changes. In the Arctic, the crowd is small and often familiar.

You see the same faces again and again.

Not only the professionals, but the community members: family who attend out of concern, out of loyalty, out of obligation, out of fear, out of curiosity. People who sit quietly in the back and already know the story before the Crown stands up to summaries it. People who recognize each other's coats. People who understand relationships that the record will never capture.

Even the accused are often familiar, not as individuals you have met personally, but as names that recur in files, as patterns that return: breaches, intoxication, violence, remorse, relapse, another breach.

The intimacy of a public system is one of the quiet shocks of circuit work. Court is public by design, but in small communities public is not an abstract principle. Public is personal. Public has a family tree.

It changes the emotional temperature of everything.

A sentencing decision does not land in a vacuum. It lands in a place where people will see each other at the store, in the hotel lobby, at the nursing station, at the arena, at the airport. Victims and accused may be related. Witnesses may be neighbors. Service providers may be friends of the family. Even professionals are not immune to the closeness. You can feel how careful everyone has to be with tone, with language, with dignity, because words spoken in court do not stay in court. They travel.

For someone in my role, the intimacy creates a particular ethical tension.

I am there to offer an opinion, sometimes written, sometimes spoken, sometimes simply guiding a decision behind the scenes. But I am also there as a visitor, carrying an authority that is both needed and potentially disruptive.

On circuit days, I learned to pay attention to how quickly a courtroom can begin to treat a person as a category.

Repeat offender.

Non-compliant.

Intoxicated.

High risk.

Breach machine.

Those phrases are efficient. They help a docket move. But they also flatten. And flattening, in a small community, has a particular cruelty: the person being flattened might be someone's cousin. Someone's son. Someone who was once the kid who played hockey. Someone who was once a quiet student. Someone who has been unwell for a long time.

The courtroom's rhythm encourages speed. Forensic psychiatry encourages caution. Circuit life demands both.

The work, then, becomes partly about timing: knowing when to speak and when not to, knowing when a clinical point will clarify, and when it will complicate in a way that serves nobody. Knowing that sometimes the most respectful thing you can do is to hold back, because the system is already heavy and your words will add weight.

There were days when the docket moved like a river in spring, fast, unstoppable, carrying everything with it.

And there were days when it stalled completely, adjournments stacking like snowdrifts, each one reasonable, each one a reminder that reason does not always produce progress.

Urgency has its own soundtrack: papers shuffling, whispered consultations, a clerk calling names, counsel moving quickly toward the bench, the judge's steady voice trying to keep structure where structure is constantly threatened. You can feel the institution trying to maintain its dignity while negotiating with realities it cannot control.

And in the middle of it all are the people whose lives are being sorted.

Circuit court days compress human complexity into short segments of time. A life becomes a summary. A history becomes a few dates. Trauma becomes "background." An illness becomes a label, if it is recognized at all.

A capacity question becomes a yes or no that does not do justice to the grey zones where most real lives are lived.

By the end of the first circuit court day, I understood something fundamental: the courtroom is not only a legal space. In the North, it is also a community space, one that carries, visibly, the intersection of justice, health, and social reality.

You leave the courthouse and you do not leave the court behind. You see its traces in the faces you pass, in the conversations you overhear, in the careful way people avoid looking too directly at each other in a hallway. The system is public. The impact is private. And the boundary between the two is thin.

That is the rhythm of circuit court days: dockets, delays, adjournments, urgency.

And the intimacy of seeing the same faces, over and over, until you understand that in the Arctic, justice is not distant.

It is close enough to touch.

CHAPTER 6

Distance, Delay, and the Meaning of "Timely Justice"

In southern cities, "timely justice" is usually discussed as a principle, something anchored in policy, statutes, and case law, measured in months and argued in courtrooms where the lights always work and the roads always exist.

In the Arctic, timely justice is not a principle first. It is a problem of physics.

Distance changes everything. Not metaphorically. Literally. Distance turns time into an obstacle course. It inserts weather between decision and action. It makes the simplest next step—an appearance, an assessment, a transfer, a treatment appointment—dependent on forces that do not care what the Criminal Code says or what the docket demands.

And so, in the North, delay is not always failure. Sometimes, delay is geography doing what geography does.

But even when delay is explainable, it is not neutral. Someone pays for it.

Often, the person who pays is the one on remand.

REMAND BY GEOGRAPHY.

There is a particular kind of custody that happens in remote settings. It does not look like a policy decision. It looks like inevitability.

A person is arrested. There are allegations. There is a bail hearing. Conditions are proposed. A plan is discussed. In a southern setting, a court may talk about treatment referrals, release plans, supervision, appointments, programs, transportation. The assumption is that the infrastructure exists, and if it does not exist, it exists somewhere nearby.

In the Arctic, the question is sometimes simpler and harsher:

Where can this person physically go?

If housing is unstable, if family relationships are strained, if the community is small and conflict is immediate, if no safe address exists, if a no-contact order effectively eliminates the only available couch, then release can become a theoretical option rather than a practical one.

And even if release is possible, the conditions required can be impossible to fulfil.

Curfews in houses where ten people share two bedrooms.

Abstinence requirements in communities where alcohol is both prohibited and pervasive.

No-contact orders in a place where you cannot avoid seeing someone at the only store, the only clinic, the only road that leads anywhere.

Mandatory counselling when the counsellor visits once a month, if the plane arrives.

When conditions are unrealistic, breaches become predictable. Predictable breaches become new charges. New charges become new remand.

And remand becomes its own kind of sentence, served not because a judge intended punishment, but because geography and scarcity silently make alternatives collapse.

This is what I began to think of as remand by geography.

A person can be "held" not only by risk, but by the absence of options. The legal language remains clean: detention is necessary, release plan is insufficient. But beneath it is a logistical truth: sometimes the system detains because it has nowhere else to place the person safely.

Forensic psychiatry enters this world with its own questions: fitness, responsibility, risk, capacity.

But those questions can become distorted when delay is baked into the environment. Symptoms worsen in custody. People decompensate under fluorescent lights and constant noise. Withdrawal happens behind bars instead of under medical care. Depression thickens in segregation. Anxiety becomes panic when you do not know when you will see your lawyer again, or whether the next court date will actually happen, or whether a flight will come.

Remand is supposed to be temporary.

In the Arctic, temporary can stretch. And stretching changes the person.

WHEN "TREATMENT" IS POSTPONED BY WEATHER

In many justice systems, "treatment" is spoken of with a kind of optimism. A referral. A program. A bed. A consultation. A plan.

In the Arctic, treatment is often spoken of with caution.

Not because people do not believe in care. They do. Everyone does: nurses, court workers, families, even officers who have seen too much to be naïve. But they know what visiting professionals learn quickly: care is not only about clinical intent. It is also about transport and timing.

Weather can cancel appointments.

Weather can postpone assessments.

Weather can prevent transfer to a hospital.

Weather can delay medication supply.

Weather can strand a patient far from supports, or strand a clinician in a hotel with a schedule that no longer matches reality.

There is a particular heartbreak to postponed treatment in forensic work. A person may finally be ready to accept help, or finally be compelled to accept help under a court order, and then the help cannot arrive because the plane cannot land.

There is also a particular danger.

Acute psychosis does not pause for wind.

Severe withdrawal does not wait for visibility to improve.

Suicidality does not follow the flight schedule.

I remember how often "we will do it next week" or "we will get them out on the next flight" was said with genuine intention, only to be undone by the simplest sentence: the flight is cancelled.

When that happens, the system improvises.

Nurses do what they can with what they have.

Guards try to keep someone safe in spaces not designed for treatment.

Court dates are moved, sometimes repeatedly, until the legal process begins to feel detached from the reality it is meant to address.

And the person at the center of it all learns something quickly: promises are fragile here, not because people are careless, but because the environment is powerful.

Treatment becomes postponed not by neglect, but by storm.

Which creates an ethical tension that is difficult to hold: we want to see the system as accountable, and it should be accountable, but we also have to acknowledge that there are days when accountability collides with aerodynamics.

THE STRANGE MATHEMATICS OF WAITING

Delay has a different emotional flavor in the North.

In southern systems, delay is frustrating. In northern systems, delay can be existential.

If court is delayed, someone remains in custody.

If a psychiatric assessment is delayed, someone may remain unmedicated, misunderstood, or misclassified.

If a transfer is delayed, someone may remain in a jail cell while sick.

If a counsellor cannot come, someone returns to the same environment without support and is then blamed for failing to change.

Waiting becomes a form of pressure. It pushes people toward despair or toward impulsivity. It strains families already living at the edge. It erodes trust in institutions that are trying, often genuinely, to do their best with what they have.

And for a visiting forensic psychiatrist, waiting carries its own unease. You are invited north to reduce uncertainty. Yet you learn that uncertainty is not just psychological. It is structural. It is meteorological. It is logistical.

You can write an opinion. You can recommend treatment. You can highlight risk and protective factors. You can propose a plan.

But you cannot command weather.

WHAT "TIMELY JUSTICE" MEANS HERE

Over time, I came to see that "timely justice" in the Arctic cannot be measured only by timelines. It has to be measured by responsiveness.

How quickly can the system pivot when plans change?

How well can it protect dignity during delay?

How safely can it hold someone who is unwell when transfer is impossible?

How realistically can it craft conditions that people can actually meet?

How thoughtfully can it use scarce resources without making scarcity itself a punishment?

The North forces the justice system to confront a truth that is usually hidden in urban abundance: time is not evenly distributed. Some people wait longer not because they deserve to wait longer, but because their lives are farther from the center.

That is the injustice inside delay.

And yet, there is also something clarifying about it. The Arctic makes visible what many systems prefer not to admit: "timely" is not just a legal standard. It is a function of infrastructure.

Roads. Planes. Housing. Clinics. Staff. Interpreters.

Without them, timeliness is a promise written on paper, easily erased by wind.

On circuit, I watched courtrooms do their best to keep pace with reality, moving dockets when they could, adjourning when they must, trying to hold urgency without surrendering fairness. I watched nurses hold care together with improvisation and stamina. I watched families absorb the costs of waiting in ways no docket ever recorded.

And I began to understand that in this place, delay is not only about time.

It is about distance.

It is about the weather.

It is about who has to pay the price when the plane does not come.

CHAPTER 7

The Community Context

You can arrive in the Arctic with a suitcase full of credentials and still understand almost nothing.

Forensic psychiatry, at its best, is supposed to be disciplined about context. We are trained to look beyond the charge, beyond the index incident, beyond the tidy summary that turns a life into a paragraph. We are trained to ask: What happened? Why now? What are the risks? What are the protections? What can realistically change?

But on circuit, context is not just a layer you add to an assessment.

Context is the assessment.

It is the air the person has been breathing for years.

In files, the community context appears as scattered details, almost footnotes:

"Lives with multiple family members."

"Unemployed."

"History of trauma."

"Alcohol involved."

"Known to police."

"Breach of conditions."

The words look familiar. They could describe people in many places. The difference here is that the words often refer to conditions that are not occasional stressors but structural facts.

HOUSING: WHEN "AN ADDRESS" IS NOT A PLAN

In many bail hearings, the conversation begins with an address.

Where will you live? With whom? How stable is it? How far is it from the complainant? Is there supervision? Is there a curfew plan?

In northern communities, "address" can be a fragile concept. Housing may be overcrowded. The meaning of "private space" may be thin. A person can be sleeping on a couch in a living room that never goes fully quiet, in a house where the temperature is controlled inside but the emotional climate is not. Families carry each other because there are no other options.

Overcrowding does more than create discomfort. It amplifies everything: conflict, stress, insomnia, relapse triggers, exposure to violence, exposure to substance use, and exposure to arguments that have nowhere to dissipate.

And when a court orders conditions that depend on space, separate bedrooms, avoidance of certain people, keeping away from triggers, or complying with a curfew, it can feel like asking someone to perform stability in an environment built on shortage.

A breach sometimes begins with nowhere to stand.

FOOD INSECURITY: THE QUIET PRESSURE THAT SHAPES BEHAVIOR

Food insecurity rarely appears in forensic reports unless someone asks directly. It is not always visible in the file. It shows up indirectly:

- Missed appointments
- Irritability and fatigue
- Medication nonadherence (because taking medication on an empty stomach feels unbearable)
- Prioritizing immediate needs over long-term plans
- Trading, borrowing, hustling, sometimes crossing legal lines

In the Arctic, food is not just expensive; it is uncertain. Even when people are resilient and resourceful, uncertainty creates a background stress that affects decision-making. Hunger sharpens impulsivity. Chronic nutritional instability erodes mood. Shame keeps people from naming it as a factor, even when it is obvious to those who have lived it.

When you see a pattern of "poor choices," you have to ask whether the person is also living under a constant arithmetic of scarcity: what can we afford today, what will we eat, what will the children have, what will run out first?

This arithmetic does not excuse harm. But it does explain why some people live closer to the edge of desperation than the file admits.

VIOLENCE EXPOSURE: WHEN "RISK" IS LEARNED EARLY

In many of the cases I encountered, violence was present long before the index offence.

Not always as perpetration first, but as exposure.

Children seeing assaults. Teenagers witnessing intoxicated rage. Homes where threats were normalized. Relationships where control was confused with love. Generations learning that escalation is how conflict gets settled when no one has ever modelled de-escalation with safety.

Violence exposure changes the nervous system. It trains people to scan for danger, to strike first, to mistrust softness, and to interpret ambiguity as threat. It can also create numbness, the kind that makes risk feel unreal until consequences arrive.

In forensic files, violence exposure is often summarized as "history of trauma." The phrase is so common it can become meaningless.

But trauma is not a decoration on the record. It is a shaping force. And when it remains untreated, it often returns as the very thing the court is trying to stop: aggression, impulsivity, substance use, dissociation, risky associations, breaches, and escalating patterns that look "criminal" but are also symptomatic.

HISTORICAL TRAUMA: THE DEEPER CURRENT

There are harms that do not begin in the individual life story. They begin earlier, through colonization, forced displacement, residential schools, family separation, cultural suppression, and systemic neglect. These harms do not stay in the past. They move forward through parenting patterns, coping strategies, grief responses, and community trust, or lack of trust, in institutions.

As a visitor, I had to hold this carefully.

It is easy to mention historical trauma as a way of sounding informed. It is much harder to let it reshape your clinical posture.

Because if you take historical trauma seriously, you cannot arrive assuming the system is trusted. You cannot assume that being asked questions by a professional is neutral. You cannot assume that a court-ordered assessment is experienced as "help." For some, it is experienced as surveillance, as judgement, as another version of being controlled by outsiders.

This matters in forensic work because the assessment itself can become part of the harm if done without humility. The questions we ask, about childhood, about violence, and about substance use, can reopen wounds, and the person may not believe the system has any right to ask or any capacity to help.

So you learn to ask differently: slower, with permission, and with clarity about why you are asking and what will happen to the answer.

HOW CONTEXT SHOWS UP AS CHARGES, BREACHES, AND ESCALATING RISK

Context is not an abstract "background." It shows up on the front page of the file.

It shows up as:

- Breaches: conditions that cannot be met in overcrowded housing or tight communities
- Assault charges: conflicts that escalate quickly in spaces where people cannot separate
- Public intoxication: coping that becomes visible because private space is limited
- Theft and mischief: survival behaviors and impulsive decisions under scarcity

- Threats: learned language of power when a person has little else that feels powerful
- Failures to appear: transportation challenges, chaotic lives, fear, shame, and disorganization

It also shows up in escalation.

A person does not start as "high risk." Often, they start as a child carrying too much. Then a teenager coping poorly. Then an adult whose coping becomes criminalized. Then a person cycling through custody, losing stability with each turn, becoming more dysregulated, more mistrustful, and more likely to reoffend—not always because they want to harm, but because their life has become a repeating pattern of rupture.

That is how risk escalates: not only through individual pathology, but through repeated exposure to instability without meaningful interruption.

THE UNCOMFORTABLE TRUTH FOR A FORENSIC VISITOR

The uncomfortable truth is that the justice system often becomes the institution that absorbs what the health and social systems could not hold.

When housing is scarce, the jail becomes the holding space.

When mental health services are thin, the courtroom becomes the triage center.

When addiction treatment is delayed, probation becomes the treatment plan, until it fails.

This does not mean people are not responsible for harm. They are. Accountability matters, especially for victims. But accountability without realism becomes performative.

In the Arctic, realism means admitting that many of the "risk factors" in our templates are not personal attributes; they are community conditions. And community conditions require community-level solutions: housing, food security, trauma-informed services, culturally grounded supports, realistic bail planning, and continuity of care that survives weather and staffing gaps.

As I continued my circuit work, I began to listen for context as carefully as I listened for symptoms. I learned to read breaches not only as rule-breaking, but as signals: this plan does not fit this life. I learned to treat "noncompliance" as a hypothesis, not a conclusion.

And above all, I learned this:

If you do not understand the community context, you will misunderstand the person.

And in forensic psychiatry, misunderstanding does not just lead to a bad report.

It can change the course of someone's life.

CHAPTER 8

Language, Interpretation, and Legal Meaning

In forensic psychiatry, words are never "just words." They become evidence. They become findings. They become conclusions that travel from an interview room into a courtroom and then into a judgment that can alter a life. In the south, I sometimes took for granted that when someone answered a question, I could at least assume we were using the same language in roughly the same way.

In the Arctic, that assumption fell apart quickly.

Here, language is not only a tool of communication. It is a boundary, a bridge, and sometimes a trap.

On circuit, interpretation was not an optional accommodation; it was the center of the work. And with interpretation came a new kind of clinical humility: the realization that the quality of your assessment can rise or fall on the translation of a single word.

THE INTERPRETER AS CO-CLINICIAN AND CO-WITNESS

The interpreter sat with us not as an accessory, but as a third presence shaping the conversation. Their job was not simply to substitute words. Their job was to carry meaning across worlds that do not align neatly.

I learned quickly that interpretation is emotionally demanding. The interpreter hears distress twice, once in the speaker's language, and once again as they recreate it in mine. They carry the weight of confidentiality in a small place where everyone is connected. They sometimes translate stories that involve people they know, families they recognize, events they have heard about long before court documents arrived.

They do this while maintaining a professional composure that most of us would struggle to hold if we were placed in the same position.

And so, from the beginning, I had to treat interpretation with respect, not performative respect, but operational respect. Pace matters. Pauses matter. Letting the interpreter finish matters. Giving space for clarification matters. A rushed interview is not just rude; it is unsafe.

TRANSLATING EMOTION

Emotion does not translate like a noun.

When a person says "I'm angry" in English, I can ask about intensity, triggers, bodily sensations, thoughts, and behavior. But in many languages, emotion may be described through physical states, through metaphors, through relational terms, or through silence that signals what words cannot safely hold.

I began to notice that people did not always label emotion directly. They might describe a tightness in the chest, a heaviness in the head, a feeling of heat, a sense of being "too full," or "not right." They might describe actions rather than feelings: "I walked out," "I stayed quiet," "I went outside," "I drank."

In a legal context, this matters because the court often wants a clean description of affect and intent.

But human beings rarely experience their inner life cleanly, and translation can make it look cleaner than it is.

Sometimes a complex emotional state becomes simplified in English, reduced to a single word like "sad" or "mad," because there is no perfect match, or because the interpreter chooses the closest practical option to keep the conversation moving. This is not an error. It is the reality of translation. But it means the clinician has to be cautious about treating translated emotion words as if they are precise psychiatric data.

I learned to ask, repeatedly and gently, "What does that mean for you?"

And to accept that sometimes the answer would come through story rather than definition.

TRANSLATING SYMPTOMS

Symptoms can also be distorted in translation.

A question like "Do you hear voices?" seems straightforward until it is not. Does the person mean external auditory hallucinations? Do they mean intrusive thoughts? Do they mean memories that feel alive? Do they mean spiritual experiences? Do they mean the inner voice of conscience? Do they mean the echo of trauma?

In forensic contexts, fitness assessments, criminal responsibility assessments, and risk assessments, these distinctions matter. A misinterpreted symptom can lead to a misdiagnosis. A misdiagnosis can lead to a legal outcome that is unjust, or an intervention that does not fit.

Even the concept of "depression" is not universal in how it is named. Some people describe it as exhaustion, as a loss of appetite, as "nothing feels good," or as "my spirit is tired." If I impose my categories too quickly, I risk turning an expression of suffering into a clinical label that the person does not recognize and may not accept.

And then there is trauma, often described in fragments, with long pauses, with sudden changes in tone. The interpreter must translate not only content but pacing, and pacing is part of meaning. A long pause can signal shame, fear, dissociation, respect, grief, or the simple fact that the person is choosing words carefully because they know those words can become legal evidence.

TRANSLATING INTENT: THE MOST DANGEROUS ZONE

In the courtroom, intent is a gravitational force.

Did you mean to do it?

Did you know what you were doing?

Did you understand it was wrong?

Were you trying to harm?

These questions can become perilous when language and culture do not align. Some people communicate indirectly. Some cultures value restraint in direct self-assertion. Some people avoid direct "yes" or "no" answers out of politeness, out of caution, or out of mistrust. Some people have learned that speaking plainly to authority can bring harm.

In that context, a simple question can produce an answer that looks clear but is not.

"YES" MAY NOT MEAN YES

In some interactions, "yes" can mean:

- "I hear you."
- "I understand your question."

- "I am being polite."
- "I want this to end."
- "I do not want conflict."
- "I am not comfortable disagreeing."

A nod can be agreement, or acknowledgment, or compliance without internal assent.

"NO" MAY NOT MEAN NO

"No" can also be complicated. It can mean:

- "I do not want to talk about that."
- "That is not how we speak about this."
- "I do not trust you yet."
- "I cannot say that here."
- "It is shameful."

And in a forensic setting, where shame and fear are common, "no" can sometimes be a protective shield rather than a factual denial.

SILENCE IS NOT EMPTY

In the Arctic, silence can be many things at once:

- Respect
- Careful consideration
- Grief
- Mistrust

- Fear of consequences
- The presence of an interpreter adding an extra step
- A culturally appropriate way to hold emotion rather than display it

Silence can also be the only safe answer when the question itself carries risk.

As a forensic psychiatrist, the worst mistake is to treat silence as data that confirms your bias.

Silence is not an answer until you understand what silence means in that room, with that person, in that community, under those circumstances.

THE RISKS OF MISUNDERSTANDING

When misunderstandings happen in clinical practice, they can lead to poor rapport, missed symptoms, or a treatment plan that fails.

In forensic work, misunderstandings can become something more serious:

- An inaccurate opinion about mental state at the time of the offence
- An incorrect conclusion about fitness or capacity
- An inflated or minimized risk assessment
- A sentencing recommendation that does not fit the person or the community
- A credibility judgment that is based on language differences rather than truthfulness

One of the most dangerous errors is confusing communication style with deception.

A person who avoids eye contact may be showing respect, not evasiveness.

A person who answers briefly may be culturally restrained, not uncooperative.

A person who nods may be polite, not consenting.

A person who pauses may be thinking, not fabricating.

In court, these differences can be misread quickly, and once misread, they can be hard to correct.

LEARNING TO ASK RESPECTFULLY

Over time, I developed a set of habits, not rigid rules, but ways of protecting meaning:

- I asked shorter questions, one at a time.
- I avoided idioms and metaphors that do not translate.
- I asked the interpreter to flag uncertainty rather than "smooth it over."
- I checked back: "Can you tell me in your own words what you understood?"
- I invited correction: "If I am misunderstanding, please tell me."
- I respected pauses as part of the conversation.
- I treated "yes" with caution and followed it with open questions.

Most importantly, I began to see that in the Arctic, interpretation is not only about language.

It is about power.

Who is allowed to speak.

Who is believed.

Whose meaning becomes "official."

Whose silence is interpreted as guilt.

A visiting forensic psychiatrist sits inside that power whether they intend to or not. The ethical task is not to pretend the power is not there, but to handle it carefully, to slow down enough to let meaning emerge rather than forcing meaning into the shape the system prefers.

Because once meaning enters a legal document, it hardens.

And in a place where everyone is connected, and where the court is both public and intimate, a hardened misunderstanding can echo for years.

That is why, on circuit, language became one of my most important clinical tools, not the language I spoke, but the language I learned to approach with humility.

To translate emotion, symptoms, and intent without flattening them.

To treat "yes," "no," and silence as invitations to understand, rather than shortcuts to certainty.

PART III

HOW CARE ACTUALLY HAPPENS

CHAPTER 9

Walking Through the Sally Port

The first time I walked through the sally port in Iqaluit, I understood, physically, what it means to cross from public space into custody.

Outside, the air was so cold it felt like it had edges. Inside, the temperature changed quickly, and with it the body's posture. Shoulders loosened. Breath softened. Eyelashes stopped freezing. The transition was abrupt, like stepping from one set of rules into another.

The sally port is not a hallway. It is a threshold with intention, a controlled pocket of space where movement is managed, not assumed. It is where the institution begins to speak in its own language: locks, pauses, procedures. It is where you learn that entry is not a right; it is a temporary permission.

The sound was the first thing that stayed with me.

Not loud, exactly, but decisive. Doors closing with a heavy finality. Clean, mechanical clicks that signal a sequence. Radio murmurs. Footsteps, boots, measured and practiced, the sound of people who spend their days moving in places where movement always matters. Even silence in custody has structure. It is not the relaxed silence of a waiting room. It is a silence that feels supervised.

Then the smell.

Institutions have a scent. The mix is difficult to name because it is not one thing. Cleaning products. Air that has been recirculated too long. The faint trace of sweat. Damp clothing drying. Industrial heat. Underneath it all, something else, an emotional smell, if such a thing exists. A smell of confinement. A smell of many anxious bodies passing through the same narrow space day after day.

I paused long enough to register the routines unfolding around me.

Routine is the architecture of jail life. It is how chaos is prevented from swallowing the place whole. Routines protect staff. They protect inmates. They protect the institution's fragile promise that order can be maintained.

But routine also has a cost. Routine can dull individuality. It can reduce people to categories: inmate, remand, escort, visitor. It can make the extraordinary ordinary.

And what struck me most was how quickly I, too, became part of the routine, as soon as I stepped inside.

I was introduced again, this time not by name alone, but by role.

Doctor. Psychiatrist. Here to assess.

In some rooms, those labels open doors. In others, they do not.

In custody, I entered as a visitor with a particular kind of authority, the kind that comes from the court's needs and the system's request for expert opinion. But I also entered with limits that were immediate and non-negotiable.

I could not decide where I would sit.

I could not decide who would escort me.

I could not decide how long the interview would be.

I could not decide what would happen if someone became agitated, or silent, or refused.

I could not decide whether the person I came to see would actually be available when I arrived.

My authority existed, but it was borrowed, conditional, and always secondary to the institution's first mandate: safety.

That is the reality of walking into jail as a visiting forensic psychiatrist. You do not arrive as the most powerful person in the room. You arrive as someone the system will accommodate, if it can, within boundaries it cannot compromise.

And so, you learn to hold your professional identity differently.

In hospitals, I am used to clinical authority being expressed through choice. I can propose, negotiate, persuade. I can often shape the environment to support a conversation: privacy, time, comfort, a sense of safety.

In jail, you work inside a space shaped for containment, not for disclosure.

The work still has to happen. But the environment sets the terms.

The staff were professional. Courteous in a way that had nothing to do with warmth and everything to do with clarity. You could feel the competence in how they moved and how they watched. Not suspicion exactly, but vigilance that has become a steady muscle.

That vigilance is not an attitude. It is a form of care.

People often misunderstand custody staff from the outside, imagining them as either harsh or indifferent. In reality, many carry a daily responsibility that few people would tolerate: keeping order among people who are frightened, angry, intoxicated, withdrawing, psychotic, grieving, or simply trapped in a life that keeps collapsing in on itself.

That day, I noticed the small gestures of routine humanity: a brief check-in, a measured tone, a refusal delivered without humiliation. The kind of professionalism that prevents escalation not through force, but through consistency.

Still, the power in the building was unmistakable.

It sat in the doors.

It sat in the pauses between movements.

It sat in the way a person's body adjusts when they are told where to stand.

It sat in the fact that my own movement, my entrance, my exit, was a privilege.

I remember thinking, briefly and uncomfortably, about how easy it was for me to leave.

That is one of the moral tensions of visiting work. You cross thresholds that others cannot cross back through. You walk into confinement with your coat on and your credentials in your pocket, and you will walk back out into open air.

The people you assess may not.

It changes how you listen, if you allow it to.

A staff member led me onward, deeper into the facility, toward the space where the interview would take place. As we moved, I became more aware of my own senses, of how the body stays alert in unfamiliar environments, how the mind scans for cues: Where are the exits? How close am I standing? How do I keep my posture calm without looking naïve?

Forensic psychiatry often requires calm in the presence of charged narratives. Jail adds another layer: calm in the presence of controlled space.

We reached the interview area, and I was reminded again that the work here is both ordinary and extraordinary.

Ordinary because people do this every day: staff, inmates, nurses, administrators. Extraordinary because the stakes can be enormous, and the human suffering is often close to the surface, even when it is masked by jokes or silence or hostility.

Before the interview began, there was a moment, a small moment, that I have come to recognize as part of the sally port experience, even when you have already passed through it.

A moment of internal recalibration.

You remind yourself: I am here to assess, not to rescue.

You remind yourself: I must be fair, not flattering.

You remind yourself: my words will travel farther than this room.

You remind yourself: this person's dignity is not optional, even here.

And you remind yourself of the visitor identity, the one that can either protect you from arrogance or expose you to it.

Because there is a seductive danger in being invited into custody spaces. A person can begin to feel important simply because doors open for them. A person can confuse access with expertise, movement with mastery.

The Arctic corrected that illusion quickly.

Walking through the sally port, I felt both the weight of being brought in to offer an opinion and the humility of realizing how little control I truly had. The institution had its own gravity, and I was briefly caught in it.

I had authority, and limits.

I had purpose, and uncertainty.

I had access, but not ownership.

And as the door closed behind me with that unmistakable sound, a sound that said, you are in now, I understood that this was where forensic psychiatry met reality. Not in courtroom arguments. Not in the elegance of diagnostic language. But here, in the controlled air of custody, where human complexity is compressed into routines, and the cost of misunderstanding can be counted in days, months, or years.

CHAPTER 10

The Interview Room

The interview room in a jail is designed to do one thing well: reduce risk.

Everything else—comfort, warmth, nuance, the slow unfolding of trust—comes second, if it comes at all. You feel that the moment you step inside. The room does not invite honesty the way a clinic office might. It invites containment.

There is a table bolted down or heavy enough not to move easily. Chairs that are functional, not forgiving. Walls that have learned to absorb noise. A door that closes with a sound that does not suggest privacy so much as control. Sometimes there is a window. Sometimes there is a camera. Often there is a sense, whether visible or not, that someone, somewhere, can see into the room.

In a hospital, you can create a therapeutic space. In a jail, you inherit a surveillance space and try to practice psychiatry inside it.

That is the work.

SAFETY PROCEDURES: THE CHOREOGRAPHY OF CONTROL

Before the patient arrives, the procedures unfold with a steady choreography.

You are escorted. You wait where you are told to wait. You do not wander. You learn quickly that "just stepping out for a minute" is not a small act here; it changes staffing, keys, sightlines, and accountability.

Someone checks the room. Someone checks the timing. Someone checks the person being brought in, searches, restraints, escort plans. There are rules about what can be brought into the room. Pens and paper can become contraband. A stethoscope can become a risk. Even a hot drink is, in the logic of custody, a potential weapon.

The staff do not do these things to humiliate the person. They do them because they have learned, often through hard experience, how quickly a situation can turn.

As a visitor, you have to respect that experience.

In forensic psychiatry, we talk about "risk factors" as abstract variables. In custody, risk is embodied and immediate. It is in how close you sit. It is in whether the door is locked. It is in whether an officer remains nearby. It is in whether the person has had bad news that morning, whether they are withdrawing, whether they are hearing voices, whether they are ashamed, whether they are angry.

Safety procedures are not an obstacle to the work. They are the conditions that make the work possible. But they also shape the work in ways that are hard to ignore.

POWER DYNAMICS: THE INVISIBLE THIRD PERSON

In a jail interview, power is always present, even when no one mentions it.

It sits in the uniform.

It sits in the keys.

It sits in the fact that one person can leave and the other cannot.

It sits in the fact that the person you are seeing may have been woken up, escorted, searched, restrained, brought to you under conditions that are not negotiated.

And then you arrive, clean coat, warm gloves, a clipboard or notebook, carrying the authority of the court's request. You may be there to assess fitness, criminal responsibility, risk, or to provide a treatment-oriented consult. Whatever the specific task, the person in custody often understands one thing clearly:

Your words will matter more than theirs.

That is the power dynamic at the heart of forensic work. In a southern outpatient clinic, the patient can walk out, refuse, choose another provider. In jail, refusal has consequences, and "choice" is narrowed.

Some people respond to that dynamic with hostility. Some with charm. Some with silence. Some with performances of compliance. Some with raw vulnerability, because they have nothing left to protect.

As a forensic psychiatrist, you learn not to take any of it at face value, not because people are inherently deceptive, but because custody conditions distort normal communication. People adapt in ways that keep them safe.

And safety, in jail, can mean looking tough. Or looking agreeable. Or looking unbothered. Or looking confused. Or saying "yes" to everything.

PRIVACY CONSTRAINTS: THE HARDEST INGREDIENT TO REPLACE

Therapeutic conversation depends on privacy.

Forensic conversation depends on privacy too, perhaps even more, because you are asking questions that can expose shame, trauma, and legal vulnerability. Yet jail interviews often provide the thinnest version of privacy available.

The person may know that officers are nearby. They may suspect the conversation is monitored. They may worry that other inmates will hear and use what is said against them later. They may fear that disclosure will travel back to family, back to community, back to the streets of a small town where anonymity does not exist.

Even if the room is technically private, it rarely feels private.

And feeling private matters.

There are things people will not say if they believe they are being watched.

There are things they will exaggerate if they believe performance will help them.

There are things they will confess too quickly if they believe confession will end the interview.

As a visitor, you have to work with what you have, and be honest about what you do not have. I learned to name the constraints directly, without dramatizing them:

"Here is what I can and cannot keep confidential."

"Here is what I am being asked to do."

"Here is how my report may be used."

"Here is what happens if you choose not to answer."

Clarity is a form of respect. It is also a way of reducing harm.

BUILDING RAPPORT UNDER SURVEILLANCE

Rapport in custody is different.

In a clinic, rapport grows through comfort and continuity. In jail, rapport grows through fairness, predictability, and tone.

The person I am seeing is often trying to answer one urgent question before they even listen to mine:

Are you here to help me, or to hurt me?

Sometimes that question is asked directly. More often, it is asked through behavior, testing, challenging, withholding.

I learned to start with small things that restore a sense of dignity:

- Introducing myself plainly
- Explaining my role without legal jargon
- Acknowledging that the setting is not comfortable
- Asking if they need water, if they are too cold, if they can hear the interpreter clearly
- Offering choices where I could: “Would you rather start with today, or with your history?”

These are minor gestures, but in a place where control has been taken away, small choices matter.

Then comes the careful work of listening.

Listening in jail is not passive. It is strategic. You listen for symptoms, yes, but you also listen for how the person is navigating power. You listen for what they avoid. You listen for when their voice changes. You listen for the difference between story and script.

A person may speak as if they are in court, because the jail has taught them to. They may speak in slogans: “I just want to go home.” “I’m not crazy.” “They set me up.” “I was drunk.” “I don’t remember.” “I’m fine.”

Behind these phrases there is often fear: fear of being judged, fear of being labelled, fear of being sent away, fear of losing face in the community, fear of losing their children, fear of being stuck indefinitely.

To build rapport, you do not bulldoze past the slogans. You treat them as doorways.

"What does home look like for you right now?"

"When you say you're fine, what does 'fine' mean in here?"

"What do you think the court misunderstands about you?"

"When you say you don't remember, is that because you were intoxicated, or because your mind shuts down under stress?"

You ask slowly, in a way that allows the person to become more than their charge.

And at the same time, you hold the forensic frame, because rapport does not mean collusion. It means creating enough safety for truth to appear, even if the truth is messy.

THE DOUBLE AUDIENCE PROBLEM

One of the strangest tensions in a jail interview is that there is often a "double audience."

The person is speaking to you, but they are also speaking to the system they imagine behind you.

They may see you as:

- A route to release
- A threat to release
- A neutral evaluator

- A tool of the Crown
- A tool of the defense
- A doctor who might finally name their suffering
- A visitor who will leave and never think about them again

That imagined audience shapes what is said.

So I learned to separate the conversation into two tracks:

1. The person's experience (symptoms, history, trauma, meaning)
2. The legal questions (intent, capacity, risk, fitness)

If you mix them too early, the interview becomes performative. If you keep them separate, you sometimes get closer to reality.

THE LIMITS THAT REMAIN

Even with good rapport, jail interviews have limits you cannot fix with skill alone.

You cannot create privacy where there is none.

You cannot offer continuity when your role is visiting.

You cannot promise that treatment will begin tomorrow when weather and staffing may decide otherwise.

You cannot promise that honesty will make the outcome better.

In fact, part of ethical rapport is refusing to make those promises.

What you can offer is something rarer in custody than most people realize: a moment of being treated as a full human being, with complexity, with context, with a story that is not only the story of the charge.

That moment does not solve the legal case.

But it can change how a person experiences the system.

And sometimes, it can change how the system sees the person.

In the interview room, under surveillance, with safety procedures humming quietly in the background, that is the narrow but meaningful space where forensic psychiatry tries to do its work: fair, careful, and human, inside a place designed for control.

CHAPTER 11

Remand: The Holding Pattern

Remand is supposed to be temporary.

That is the theory.

In practice, especially in the Arctic, remand can become a holding pattern that lasts long enough to change a person. It is custody without conclusion. Time served without sentence. Waiting as a condition of life.

On circuit, I met people who spoke about remand the way travelers speak about being stranded in an airport during a storm: you are not going anywhere, and no one can tell you when you will.

The difference is that in remand, the storm is not outside the building. The storm is inside the mind.

WITHDRAWAL: THE BODY'S REVOLT

Withdrawal is rarely poetic. It is physical misery, often layered with shame.

In some cases, it begins within hours of arrest: sweating, tremors, nausea, diarrhea, headache, muscle pain, anxiety that crawls under the skin. In others, it arrives after the first night, when the person realizes that the substance they used to regulate their nervous system is no longer available.

In the files, this might be summarized in a line: "appeared intoxicated," "history of substance use," "detox in custody."

But in the jail, it looks like a person trying to sleep and failing, trying to eat and gagging, trying to hold dignity while their body betrays them.

Withdrawal also alters mental state. Anxiety spikes. Irritability becomes rage. Depressive thoughts deepen. Paranoia intensifies. For some, especially those with trauma histories, withdrawal strips away the numbing layer that allowed them to function and exposes raw memory and panic.

In a place with limited medical resources, withdrawal can become more than discomfort. It can become danger.

And it can become the first step in deterioration that the system later labels as "behavior."

INSOMNIA: THE SLOW EROSION

If withdrawal is the body's revolt, insomnia is the mind's erosion.

Sleep in remand is not sleep; it is interruption.

Doors. Lights. Checks. Noise. The anxiety of being watched. The uncertainty of what tomorrow holds. The constant small frictions of living in a confined space with people you did not choose.

For people already prone to depression, anxiety, psychosis, or trauma-related hyperarousal, insomnia is gasoline.

I saw how quickly sleep deprivation can mimic psychiatric illness and worsen existing illness. A person who was irritable becomes explosive. A person who was paranoid becomes convinced. A person who was depressed becomes suicidal. A person who was stable becomes disorganized.

In forensic assessments, we often ask, "When did the symptoms start?" In remand, symptoms can start after three nights of poor sleep.

And then they begin to look like who the person is, rather than what the person is enduring.

FEAR: THE CONSTANT UNDERCURRENT

There is a fear in remand that is not always spoken.

Sometimes it is fear of violence, fear of other inmates, fear of conflict, fear of being targeted.

Sometimes it is fear of shame, fear that family will find out, fear that children will be taken, fear that community will talk.

Sometimes it is fear of the system, fear that you will be forgotten, that your lawyer will not come, that court will be postponed, that your case will be decided without you understanding what is happening.

And sometimes it is the deepest fear: fear that this holding pattern is not temporary at all, but the beginning of a life lived in cycles, arrest, remand, release, breach, remand again.

Fear changes how people present. It can make them aggressive, because aggression feels protective. It can make them compliant, because compliance feels safer. It can make them silent, because silence feels like survival.

As a visiting forensic psychiatrist, you have to see fear even when it comes disguised as attitude.

BOREDOM: THE MISUNDERSTOOD ACCELERANT

Boredom sounds harmless until you see what it does in custody.

Remand is often a place of waiting with very little structure. People who have lived chaotic lives sometimes come into custody and lose even the chaotic routines they had: their streets, their friends, their substances, their coping rituals, their distractions.

The mind turns inward. For some, that is unbearable.

Boredom becomes agitation. Agitation becomes conflict. Conflict becomes segregation. Segregation becomes deterioration.

It is not boredom as laziness. It is boredom as sensory and relational deprivation, a kind of starvation that makes people restless, irritable, and impulsive.

I began to see boredom as an accelerant for symptoms: it amplifies rumination, amplifies cravings, amplifies paranoia, amplifies hopelessness. It also amplifies "acting out," because sometimes an incident is the only way a person feels anything shift in a day that otherwise feels frozen.

WHEN MINOR CHARGES BECOME MAJOR DETERIORATION

One of the most troubling patterns I observed was how quickly a minor legal matter could become a major clinical crisis once remand entered the picture.

A person comes in on a relatively minor charge: mischief, theft under a certain amount, failure to comply, a breach that would look "manageable" in a system with supports.

If the person is housed, stable, and sober, the case might resolve quickly. But in the Arctic, those conditions cannot be assumed.

A person held on remand for a minor matter may deteriorate because:

- Their medications are interrupted or unavailable
- Withdrawal is unmanaged or partially managed
- Sleep is fragmented
- Anxiety escalates in confinement
- Trauma symptoms intensify without coping resources

- Court delays stretch the timeline
- Shame and fear cut them off from family support
- They lose their housing while in custody
- They lose their job or income
- Their relationships rupture

By the time the next court date comes, if it comes, the person is no longer the person who was arrested.

They are thinner, more agitated, more depressed, more paranoid, more hopeless. Sometimes they are suicidal. Sometimes they are aggressive. Sometimes they are so disorganized that fitness becomes a question. Sometimes they commit new incidents inside custody: threats, assaults, property damage, behaviors that become new charges, widening the legal net.

This is how a minor charge becomes a major deterioration.

Not because the person suddenly "got worse" in a vacuum, but because the holding pattern itself became pathogenic.

Remand can function like a slow toxin for vulnerable minds.

THE ARCTIC MULTIPLIER

In the Arctic, all of this is intensified by distance.

If a person becomes acutely unwell, transfer to a hospital may not be immediate. Weather may delay it. Staffing may delay it. The lack of local psychiatric beds may make it impossible. The person may remain in a setting not designed for treatment, managed by staff who do their best but cannot provide what a hospital provides.

And the person knows it. They know that help is far. They know that time is uncertain. They know that they are not simply waiting for their case; they are waiting for the system to have the capacity to move.

That knowledge can turn anxiety into despair.

WHAT I LEARNED TO WATCH FOR

Over time, I began to treat remand not as neutral custody, but as a clinically meaningful environment with predictable risks.

I watched for withdrawal masquerading as aggression.

I watched for insomnia masquerading as psychosis.

I watched for fear masquerading as defiance.

I watched for boredom masquerading as "behavioral problems."

And I watched for the quiet forms of deterioration that do not draw attention until it is too late: the person who stops eating, the person who stops talking, the person who gives away their belongings, the person who says they are "fine" with a flatness that feels like absence.

Remand is often described as a holding pattern, and the phrase is accurate, but incomplete.

A holding pattern implies that the plane is stable, simply waiting to land.

For many people in custody, the holding pattern is not stable at all.

It is a slow descent.

And the tragedy is that by the time the system is ready to "resolve" the minor charge, the person may have become a much bigger problem, clinically, legally, and humanly, than they ever needed to be.

That is the hidden cost of remand.

Not just days behind a door.

But the deterioration that happens while everyone is waiting.

CHAPTER 12

Segregation, Decompensation, and the Thin Line

There is a point in custody where the system stops pretending it is holding someone temporarily and begins, instead, to contain them.

That point is often segregation.

The word is clinical in its blandness, segregation, as if it were simply an administrative arrangement, a placement decision, a logistical solution. But what it means in lived reality is something harsher: separation as a response to fear, risk, and overwhelm. A door that closes not only on a person's body, but on their access to others, the very thing that often keeps the mind from collapsing.

In the Arctic, segregation carries additional weight because alternatives are scarce. There may be no dedicated psychiatric unit nearby, no rapid transfer, no specialized team on standby. Sometimes there is not even enough staff to provide the kind of observation that would feel humane. And when you combine confinement with crisis, the line between "management" and "treatment" becomes painfully thin.

AGITATION: WHEN THE NERVOUS SYSTEM CATCHES FIRE

Agitation in remand is rarely random. It has a logic, even when it looks chaotic.

Sometimes it begins with withdrawal, an autonomic storm, a body searching for the substance it relied on to regulate itself. Sometimes it begins with insomnia, days of fragmented sleep turning irritability into rage. Sometimes it begins with fear, fear of other inmates, fear of shame, fear of being forgotten, fear of what the court will do. Sometimes it begins with trauma, the sudden return of memories when numbing has been stripped away.

In custody, agitation is often treated as a behavioral problem. That is understandable; agitation can become dangerous quickly. Staff have to protect everyone in the building. But agitation is also often a clinical signal: the nervous system is overloaded and the person's capacity to self-regulate is failing.

The challenge is that custody environments are not designed to reduce arousal. They are designed to reduce movement.

A person who is agitated needs space, calm, dignity, predictable communication, and often medical stabilization. In jail, what they often receive is the opposite: noise, control, urgency, and the emotional charge of being watched.

If you want to understand why decompensation happens in custody, begin there.

SELF-HARM: THE LANGUAGE OF DESPERATION

I learned early and uncomfortably that some people express despair through actions rather than words. In jail, this is not always dramatic. Sometimes it is subtle, quiet signals, small changes, a flattening of voice, a withdrawal from routine. Sometimes it is more overt: a person trying to communicate unbearable distress in the only way they believe the system will recognize.

In a resource-rich setting, that moment might trigger a multidisciplinary response: rapid psychiatric review, therapeutic containment, safety planning, medication adjustments, and, importantly, a sense that the person will not be left alone with their terror.

In a resource-scarce setting, that same moment can trigger something else: placement decisions.

Where can we put them that is safest right now?

And too often, "safest" gets translated into "most controlled."

Segregation becomes the answer, not because anyone thinks it is therapeutic, but because it feels like the only environment where immediate harm can be prevented with the staff and space available.

That is one of the cruel paradoxes of custody mental health: the person most in need of human connection can end up in the place where connection is thinnest.

PSYCHOSIS: THE SYSTEM'S HARDEST TEST

Psychosis in custody is a test of the entire institution.

A person hearing voices, terrified by persecutory beliefs, disorganized, or responding to internal stimuli may not follow instructions. They may shout, pace, refuse food, refuse medication, refuse to come out, refuse to go back in. They may interpret staff actions as threats. They may believe the institution is conspiring against them. They may misread ordinary procedures as punishment.

From the outside, it can look like defiance.

From the inside, it can be pure fear.

In the Arctic, where transfers can be delayed by weather and psychiatric beds can be far away, a person in acute psychosis may remain in custody longer than anyone would want. Staff then face an impossible task: maintain safety in an environment not built for treatment, often with limited clinical support, and with thc knowledge that what is needed, specialized psychiatric care, may not arrive quickly.

Psychosis exposes the thinness of the line between correctional care and clinical care. It forces the question the system tries to avoid:

Are we managing risk, or are we treating illness?

Most days, the honest answer is: we are managing, because treatment is not fully available.

RESTRAINT DECISIONS: THE MOMENT EVERYONE DREADS

Restraint, physical or chemical, is where ethics stop being academic.

No one who has worked in custody wants to restrain someone. The decision is heavy because it carries risks: physical injury, trauma reinforcement, humiliation, and the moral weight of using force against a person who may already have a long history of being harmed.

And yet, there are moments when staff feel they have no choice. When a person is at imminent risk of hurting themselves or someone else. When de-escalation has failed. When time is measured in seconds, not minutes.

As a visiting forensic psychiatrist, I was not always present at those moments, but I encountered their aftermath: people shaken, staff exhausted, the emotional residue thick in the air. Restraints are rarely a clean solution. They are an emergency measure, and emergencies leave marks.

What stayed with me most was how often the decision arose not from malice but from scarcity:

- Scarcity of space.
- Scarcity of staff.

- Scarcity of clinical alternatives.
- Scarcity of time.

In a system under strain, restraint can become the last tool standing.

That is not an excuse. It is a warning.

THE ETHICAL TENSION: "MANAGE" VERSUS "TREAT"

In the language of forensic systems, "manage" is often framed as responsible: manage risk, manage behavior, manage safety.

In the language of medicine, "treat" is the moral anchor: treat suffering, treat illness, treat the person.

In custody, these imperatives collide.

The institution's primary mandate is safety: safety of staff, safety of inmates, safety of the public. That mandate shapes every decision. And yet, the individuals inside are human beings with illnesses, trauma histories, addictions, grief, and despair.

So the question becomes not whether to manage or treat, but how to hold both without losing your integrity.

I found myself asking repeatedly:

- Are we containing a crisis, or prolonging it?
- Are we preventing harm today while increasing harm tomorrow?
- Are we responding to illness as illness, or mislabeling it as misconduct?
- Are we using the tools we have because they are right, or because they are the only ones available?

The Arctic makes these questions sharper because the usual escape routes—transfer, specialized programs, rapid consultation—are unreliable. Weather can turn “tomorrow” into “next week.” Staffing can turn “observation” into “checks when we can.” Geography can turn “hospital care” into “waiting in custody.”

When resources are scarce, ethical practice requires an even stricter commitment to honesty: naming what is happening, naming what is missing, and refusing to pretend that containment is treatment simply because it is all we can offer.

THE THIN LINE, WALKED DAILY

The staff in northern jails—guards, nurses, administrators—walk this thin line daily. They do it with professionalism, fatigue, and often a kind of quiet moral courage that does not get recognized. They are asked to be both firm and humane, both vigilant and compassionate, in an environment that rewards control more easily than it rewards care.

And the people in custody walk the line too, between coping and collapse, between anger and despair, between survival strategies and self-destruction.

As a visitor, I walked that line differently. I came in, assessed, recommended, documented. I carried the privilege of leaving.

But I could not ignore the moral discomfort of seeing what happens when human suffering meets institutional scarcity. The discomfort was not an abstract critique of the system; it was personal. It lived in the faces of people who were unraveling behind a door and in the tired eyes of staff who wanted more options than they had.

Segregation, decompensation, restraint, the thin line is where forensic psychiatry stops being theory and becomes reality.

Not the reality of court language.

The reality of human beings in crisis, contained by necessity, and the constant ethical pressure to ensure that "management" never becomes a substitute for compassion, or an excuse to forget that treatment is what we owe, even when we cannot fully deliver it.

In the Arctic, the line is thin.

And every day, someone has to decide how to walk it.

CHAPTER 13

Medication in Custody

Medication in custody is where clinical ideals meet institutional reality.

In southern practice, prescribing often assumes a web of supports: pharmacies with full inventories, labs that can be ordered and resulted quickly, ECGs that can be arranged, follow-up appointments that can be scheduled, community teams that can monitor adherence, families who can support routines, and, crucially, choices. If a medication does not fit, there are alternatives. If side effects emerge, you can pivot.

In a northern jail, prescribing begins with a different set of questions:

- What do we actually have?
- What can we safely monitor?
- What can we deliver consistently?
- What will happen when this person is transferred or released, often suddenly?

Medication becomes less like selecting the "best" option and more like selecting the most workable option under constraints.

FORMULARIES: THE TYRANNY OF THE AVAILABLE

The custody formulary is a practical document, but it carries enormous clinical consequences. It determines what can be offered easily, what requires special ordering, and what is simply not possible.

In the Arctic, formularies are shaped not only by budget but by logistics. Medications arrive through a supply chain that can be interrupted by weather, delayed by flights, complicated by storage requirements, and constrained by staffing. Even when a medication is technically "available," it may not be consistently available.

As a visiting forensic psychiatrist, I learned to ask early, not just about diagnosis and symptoms, but about the medication reality:

- Which antipsychotics are reliably stocked?
- Which antidepressants are on hand?
- What options exist for withdrawal management?
- What is the process for non-formulary requests?
- How long does it take for a special order to arrive, when it arrives?

These are not administrative details; they are clinical determinants. A treatment plan that cannot be supplied is not a plan. It is wishful thinking.

So the art becomes choosing what will survive the environment. Sometimes that means prescribing older medications because they are stocked and familiar, even if newer ones might be preferable in an ideal world. Sometimes it means choosing a regimen with fewer monitoring requirements because monitoring is not feasible. Sometimes it means settling for "good enough to stabilize" rather than "optimal for long-term recovery."

This is not cynicism. It is triage.

MONITORING CHALLENGES: MEDICINE WITHOUT ITS USUAL SAFETY NET

Monitoring is where custody medicine can become ethically tense.

Many psychiatric medications require some form of follow-up: metabolic monitoring for antipsychotics, ECG consideration for QT-prolonging agents, lab checks for certain mood stabilizers, careful titration, and side effect surveillance. In a jail, especially a remote one, those systems may exist in partial form, dependent on staff capacity and timing.

The challenge is not that staff do not care. The challenge is that the system is stretched. A nurse may be covering multiple roles. Medical visits may be limited. Lab access may be intermittent. Transport to a facility capable of certain investigations may not be immediate. And when someone is in remand, there is the constant unpredictability of movement: a court decision, a transfer, a release.

This creates a prescribing dilemma: Do you start a medication that could meaningfully help, knowing monitoring might be imperfect? Or do you hold back, leaving the person symptomatic, because the ideal monitoring pathway is not available?

In urban settings, we rarely have to hold this dilemma so sharply. In the Arctic, it is part of routine practice.

When monitoring is limited, the clinician's responsibility becomes even more deliberate: choose simpler regimens when possible, start low and go slow, document clearly, communicate with nursing, and prioritize safety without letting fear of imperfection become inertia.

DIVERSION: WHEN PILLS BECOME CURRENCY

In custody, diversion is not theoretical. It is a daily concern.

Some medications have value beyond their therapeutic purpose. They can be traded, hoarded, used to alter consciousness, or used as leverage. Even benign-seeming medications can become part of the informal economy of a jail.

This forces a second layer of clinical thinking: not only what is indicated, but what is safe to dispense in this environment. Diversion concerns can lead to restrictions, crushing medications, supervised administration, limiting PRN use, or avoiding certain agents altogether. These practices can feel harsh to patients, especially those who have never experienced custody medicine. They may interpret supervision as mistrust, and mistrust can erode rapport.

But diversion controls exist because harm is real: overdoses, coercion, conflict, and black-market dynamics that create instability. In a small facility, a single diverted medication can ripple across the unit.

Forensic psychiatry sits awkwardly here. Our duty is to the patient, but we must also recognize that the environment is not neutral. A medication choice can influence not only symptoms but safety for others.

This is one of the quiet ways custody turns medicine into ethics.

CONTINUITY: THE FRAGILE BRIDGE ACROSS TRANSFERS AND RELEASES

If formularies and diversion are the daily challenges, continuity is the long-term one.

People in remand move. They are transferred between facilities. They are released suddenly. They return to the community, sometimes with no notice, sometimes without a follow-up appointment, sometimes without a stable place to sleep that night.

Medication continuity across these transitions is one of the most important and most vulnerable parts of care. A person stabilized on an antipsychotic can relapse quickly if it is stopped. A person started on an antidepressant can discontinue prematurely, experiencing withdrawal effects or a rebound in symptoms. A person prescribed sedatives or withdrawal management can be left vulnerable if the regimen is interrupted abruptly. A person discharged without a supply can simply run out, especially in communities where pharmacies are limited and refill processes are complex.

The consequences show up in the justice system again:

- Relapse → crisis → police involvement
- Missed appointments → breach of conditions
- Decompensation → new charges
- Destabilization → re-remand

Continuity failures are not always visible as "medical errors." They often present as "behavioral problems" or "reoffending." But underneath, the thread is clinical instability, sometimes preventable, sometimes inevitable.

As a visiting psychiatrist, I learned to treat discharge and transfer planning as part of the prescription itself.

Not: "Start medication."

But: "Start medication, and ensure it can follow the person."

That meant asking practical questions:

- Who will hold the medication list when the person leaves?
- Will the nursing station know?
- Does the person have a family member who can support adherence?
- Is there a follow-up appointment scheduled, or at least requested?
- Is there a bridging supply available?

- Is the person being released to a place where medication storage is safe?

In a resource-rich system, these questions are often delegated. In the Arctic, they are too important to assume.

THE DEEPER DILEMMA: WHAT DOES "CARE" MEAN IN CUSTODY?

Medication in custody forces a clinician to confront a deeper issue: in many cases, the jail is providing the most consistent point of contact a person has had with health care in a long time.

That is not what jails are for. And yet, it becomes true. Some people are assessed for the first time while on remand. Some receive their first stable medication regimen in custody. Some disclose trauma or psychosis for the first time in a setting that is not designed for healing.

This creates a bittersweet reality: Custody can be the first place where someone's illness is named and treated, and also the place where treatment is most fragile and most constrained.

I came to see custody prescribing as a form of realism with compassion: you do what you can with what you have, you try to stabilize without creating new harms, and you pay relentless attention to continuity, because continuity is where the gains are kept or lost.

In the Arctic, medications are not just molecules in a blister pack.

They are a promise the system makes to the person.

And every transfer, every release, every storm that delays supply tests whether that promise can hold.

PART IV

CORE FORENSIC WORK ON THE CIRCUIT

CHAPTER 14

Fitness to Stand Trial

Fitness sounds like a simple word until you hear it in a courtroom.

It is not fitness as in health or strength. It is not even fitness as in "wellness." In the justice system, fitness to stand trial is a narrow question with wide consequences: Is this person able to participate in their own defense in a basic, meaningful way?

On circuit, that question arrived again and again, sometimes as a formal referral, sometimes as a quiet concern raised in a hallway, sometimes as a judge pausing mid-docket because something about the accused person's presentation did not fit the script of court.

The challenge in the Arctic is that the question does not arrive in a vacuum. It arrives wrapped in language barriers, interrupted schooling, cognitive limitations, trauma histories, substance withdrawal, and the fatigue of remand. It arrives in a setting where "assessment" is possible, but "restoration" is often not.

COMPETENCIES IN PLAIN LANGUAGE

When I explain fitness, I start with plain language, because plain language is the only honest place to begin.

Fitness generally comes down to three core abilities:

1. **Understanding what is happening in court.**
   Not the legal theory, but the basics: Who is the judge? Who is the Crown? Who is defense counsel? What is this hearing for? What does "plea," "bail," "trial," or "sentencing" mean in simple terms?

2. **Understanding the possible outcomes.**
   Again, not in detail, but enough to grasp that decisions have consequences: custody, conditions, fines, orders, restrictions, and sometimes long-term impacts.

3. **Being able to communicate with their lawyer.**
   Not eloquently. Not strategically. But meaningfully: Can they tell their lawyer what happened? Can they answer questions? Can they give instructions? Can they follow basic advice? Can they ask for clarification when confused?

Fitness is not a test of intelligence. It is not a test of education. It is not a test of whether someone makes "good decisions." A person can be mentally ill and still be fit. A person can be difficult and still be fit. A person can be distressed and still be fit.

Fitness is about a minimum threshold of participation.

On paper, it sounds tidy. In real life, especially on circuit, it rarely is.

WHEN COGNITIVE LIMITS, LANGUAGE, AND EDUCATION BLUR THE PICTURE

In southern settings, you can sometimes separate the variables. You can take your time. You can do collateral interviews. You can arrange neuropsychological testing. You can observe over days. You can revisit questions when the person is sober and rested.

In the Arctic, time is thinner, and the variables stack.

Cognitive Limits

Some people arrive at court with long-standing cognitive challenges: developmental delay, fetal alcohol spectrum disorder, acquired brain injury, chronic effects of substance use, or untreated learning disorders. In a file, these are often absent or reduced to vague phrases, such as "limited functioning," "poor insight," or "concrete thinking." In court, they can look like confusion, passivity, or nodding without comprehension.

The risk here is misinterpretation in both directions:

- Mistaking cognitive limitation for defiance ("He is not answering because he won't")
- Mistaking anxious compliance for understanding ("He says yes, so he must get it")

In small northern communities, people may have learned to survive institutions by appearing agreeable. They nod. They say "yes." They repeat phrases they have heard before. They smile at the right moments. They do what they are told.

That can look like fitness. It can also be camouflage.

Language

When an accused person speaks through an interpreter, the fitness question becomes more complex. Not because interpreters are not skilled—many are exceptional—but because legal meaning is brittle. Words like "guilty," "not guilty," "adjournment," "conditions," "undertaking," "probation," "remand," and "trial" are not just vocabulary. They are concepts, and concepts travel unevenly across languages.

I learned to avoid asking, "Do you understand?" because it invites politeness.

Instead, I ask:

- "Tell me what you think will happen today."
- "Explain to me what your lawyer does."
- "If the judge asks you a question, what should you do?"
- "What does it mean to say 'not guilty'?"
- "What are the rules you have to follow if you are released?"

Then I listen for structure, not perfection.

If the person can explain the basic roles and the basic stakes in their own words, even with gaps, they are often fit. If they cannot, the question remains open.

Education

Education complicates fitness in a quieter way.

Some people have had interrupted schooling. Some have grown up with little exposure to formal institutions. Some have never sat in a courtroom until the day the system expects them to make decisions that will shape their future.

That does not make them unfit.

But it means the system may confuse unfamiliarity with incapacity, or, worse, may treat unfamiliarity as indifference.

Sometimes what a person needs is not a psychiatric label, but explanation and time. Sometimes they are fit, but the court process is moving too fast for their nervous system to keep up.

The Arctic Overlay

And then you add the Arctic overlay: fatigue from disrupted sleep, stress from custody, withdrawal symptoms, hunger, shame, grief, fear, and the oppressive uncertainty of whether the next court date will even happen as planned.

Fitness is assessed in a snapshot. But in the North, the snapshot is often taken in poor lighting.

RESTORING FITNESS WHEN THERE IS NO LOCAL PROGRAM

In many regions, "unfit" has a pathway. There are structured fitness restoration programs, secure hospital units, specialized teams, and legal processes that move a person from custody to treatment and back again once capacity returns.

On circuit, the hardest part is what happens when the person is likely unfit, but the local system does not have a clear restoration infrastructure.

You can name the problem. But can the system treat it?

This is where the ethical tension becomes real. Declaring someone unfit is not a kindness if the result is prolonged limbo, extended custody, repeated delays, transfers far from home, and the slow erosion of whatever stability remains. And yet, proceeding when someone is truly unfit is unjust.

So you end up working in a space where your role is both clinical and practical: not only to assess, but to help the system understand what is feasible.

Sometimes fitness restoration is pharmacological: stabilizing psychosis, reducing severe mania, treating delirium, managing withdrawal.

Sometimes it is educational: repeating information, using plain language, ensuring the person truly understands roles and choices.

Sometimes it is environmental: sleep, food, reduced chaos, basic dignity, things that should be assumed but often are not.

But in the Arctic, the same obstacle returns: distance. If the person needs hospital-level treatment, they may need to be transferred south. Transfers are delayed by weather. Beds are limited. The person leaves their community, their supports, their language. Their distress can worsen simply from dislocation.

I began to see that "restoration" in this context is often less a program and more a fragile bridge built out of phone calls, nursing ingenuity, cautious prescribing, and repeated explanation, done inside a custody environment that was never designed for treatment.

THE HUMAN COST OF GETTING IT WRONG

Fitness is a legal concept, but the consequences are deeply human.

If we decide a person is fit when they are not, the trial process becomes performance. The person appears present, but they are not participating. They may plead without understanding. They may accept conditions they cannot follow. They may agree just to end the discomfort of court.

If we decide a person is unfit when they are fit, we can trap them in a different kind of holding pattern, one that can last longer than the sentence they might have received.

That is why, on circuit, fitness assessments require more than diagnostic skill. They require humility about what you are seeing and what you are not seeing, and a disciplined resistance to shortcuts.

I learned to treat the question of fitness the way you treat ice: test it carefully, step slowly, and never assume it will hold simply because it looks solid.

Because in the Arctic, the courtroom moves on urgency. But fitness, true fitness, demands patience.

CHAPTER 15

Criminal Responsibility and Mental Disorder

There are moments in forensic psychiatry when the room gets quieter, even if no one says anything.

The question of criminal responsibility has that effect. It is not simply a clinical question, and it is not simply a legal question. It is a question that sits at the boundary of both and asks something that human beings have argued about for centuries in different languages: when does illness change what someone is accountable for?

On circuit, that question carried extra weight because the Arctic compresses so many risk factors into a small social space. People live close to one another, histories overlap, resources are thin, and trauma is often not a footnote, it is a recurring theme. Add intoxication, sleep deprivation, grief, and poverty, and the line between illness and circumstance can look blurred.

But the legal standard is not blurred. The law asks for a specific kind of analysis, and the psychiatrist is invited to translate clinical reality into legal meaning without pretending the translation is simple.

THE CLINICAL PROBLEM INSIDE THE LEGAL QUESTION

Criminal responsibility assessments often begin with an event, an offence, and the legal system's need to understand the person's mental state at the time.

That time frame matters.

The question is not "Does this person have a mental disorder?" Many people do. The question is "Did a mental disorder significantly impair their ability to understand the nature and quality of the act, or to know it was wrong?"

In practice, this becomes an exercise in reconstructing a mind in a moment, often with imperfect information, often long after the fact, often through accounts shaped by fear, shame, or strategy.

In the Arctic, the reconstruction is complicated by language, by fewer collateral sources, by delays, and by the sheer density of context.

So the work becomes careful and, at times, uncomfortable. You are trying to separate what was driven by illness from what was driven by the environment, while accepting that environment can also create illness.

PSYCHOSIS: WHEN REALITY IS NOT SHARED

When psychosis is present, the analysis can become both clearer and more complex.

Clearer because acute psychosis can profoundly distort perception and judgment. A person may act under delusions or hallucinations that make their behavior internally logical even if it appears irrational to everyone else.

More complex because not every odd belief is psychosis, and not every psychosis is obvious.

In some cases, the signs are unmistakable: paranoid delusions, command hallucinations, disorganized thinking, responding to unseen stimuli, a narrative that cannot be anchored in shared reality. In those cases, the forensic question becomes: was the offence directly shaped by psychotic experience?

But in other cases, psychosis is partial or intermittent. A person may be psychotic and also intoxicated. They may be psychotic and also angry. They may be psychotic and also caught in a conflict that is real. They may have been psychotic at baseline but not acutely psychotic at the time of the offence.

And then there is trauma, which can mimic psychosis in some ways: hypervigilance, intrusive experiences, dissociation, misinterpretation of threats, without meeting criteria for a primary psychotic disorder.

So psychosis is not a shortcut to a conclusion. It is a hypothesis that has to be tested against chronology, consistency, collateral information, and functional evidence.

- What did the person do before the offence?
- What did they do after?
- Were there signs of planning?
- Were there attempts to avoid detection?
- Did they express confusion or conviction?
- Did their account remain stable over time, or shift with what they learned about the case?

These questions do not prove criminal responsibility or lack of it. But they help you understand how the person's mind was operating in the moment.

INTOXICATION: THE LOUD CONFOUNDER

Intoxication is one of the most common and most confusing features of northern forensic cases.

Alcohol and other substances appear repeatedly in the narratives: as triggers, as coping tools, as accelerants, as the setting in which offences occur. Intoxication can produce disinhibition, memory gaps, emotional volatility, and poor judgment. It can also worsen underlying psychiatric conditions, especially psychosis and trauma-related dysregulation.

But intoxication is not the same as mental disorder in the legal sense, at least not automatically. This is where forensic psychiatry must resist simplistic explanations.

It is tempting to say, "They were drunk, therefore they did not know what they were doing." That is rarely accurate.

It is also tempting to say, "They were drunk, therefore this is purely behavioral." That is also rarely accurate.

The truth is often layered. Intoxication can be both voluntary and compulsive, both a choice and a symptom of addiction, both a social pattern and a psychiatric vulnerability. In the Arctic, intoxication often sits on top of trauma, grief, boredom, and scarcity. It is a chemistry problem and a social problem and a mental health problem all at once.

So the key task becomes distinguishing between:

- Intoxication as disinhibition (the person's baseline values and impulses amplified)
- Intoxication as delirium-like confusion (rare but possible)
- Intoxication as a trigger for psychosis (substance-induced psychosis)
- Intoxication as part of an enduring substance use disorder (a chronic condition that changes brain function and behavior over time)

Each has different implications for clinical interpretation and legal framing.

NEUROCOGNITIVE DISORDER: WHEN IMPAIRMENT LOOKS LIKE "ATTITUDE"

Some of the hardest cases involved neurocognitive vulnerabilities, developmental delay, acquired brain injury, fetal alcohol spectrum disorder, or early cognitive decline.

In court, neurocognitive impairment can be misunderstood as stubbornness. In custody, it can be misunderstood as noncompliance. In the community, it can lead to repeated conflict because the person cannot learn from consequences in the way the system expects.

In criminal responsibility analyses, neurocognitive impairment rarely produces dramatic psychotic distortion, but it can reduce judgment, impulse control, and the ability to foresee consequences. It can make a person vulnerable to being led. It can make them respond aggressively to confusion. It can make them misinterpret social cues.

It also complicates intent. A person may know something is "wrong" in a general sense but lack the executive capacity to inhibit the behavior in the moment, especially under intoxication or stress.

This is where the law and psychiatry sometimes strain against each other. The law tends to prefer crisp categories. Neurocognitive realities often live in gradients.

TRAUMA: THE INVISIBLE ENGINE

Trauma is not a diagnosis that automatically changes criminal responsibility. But trauma can shape behavior in ways that are clinically meaningful and legally relevant.

Trauma can lead to hyperarousal, a hair-trigger startle response, dissociation, emotional numbing, and a perception of threat where others see ambiguity. Trauma can create survival-oriented reactions, fight, flight, or freeze, that bypass reflective thought.

In intimate partner violence contexts, trauma can intersect with coercion and control. In community violence contexts, trauma can normalize aggression as protection. In childhood trauma contexts, trauma can impair the development of emotional regulation and attachment, leaving the person less able to manage conflict without escalation.

The forensic task is not to excuse harm through trauma. It is to understand whether trauma-related symptoms meaningfully altered perception and capacity at the time, and to document this carefully without turning it into a blanket explanation.

ILLNESS-DRIVEN ACTS VERSUS CONTEXT-DRIVEN ACTS

This distinction, illness-driven versus context-driven, sounds neat until you try to apply it to real life. Many acts are both.

A person with psychosis may be living in an environment of chronic threat and conflict. A person with trauma may be intoxicated. A person with cognitive impairment may be manipulated by others. A person may act aggressively because of paranoia and because a real argument is happening in a crowded house. Context and illness do not take turns; they overlap.

Still, the meaningful and legally relevant forensic role demands disciplined thinking:

- **Illness-driven** suggests that symptoms significantly shaped the act, such as delusions, hallucinations, gross disorganization, profound cognitive impairment, severe mood symptoms, or delirium-like confusion.

- **Context-driven** suggests that the act was primarily shaped by interpersonal conflict, social dynamics, intoxication-related disinhibition, opportunism, desperation, or learned behavior, without evidence that psychiatric symptoms were the primary driver.

The key is not to moralize either category. Context-driven does not mean a bad person. Illness-driven does not mean a good person. Both can involve harm. Both can involve suffering. Both deserve accountability and care in different proportions.

The work is to avoid two easy errors:

1. Over-medicalizing context, turning poverty, scarcity, grief, and conflict into diagnoses.
2. Under-recognizing illness, treating psychosis, neurocognitive impairment, and trauma symptoms as just behavior.

In the Arctic, both errors are tempting because the context is heavy and the suffering is widespread. It becomes easy to say, "Everyone has trauma, so this is normal." Or to say, "This is all trauma, so nothing is responsibility." Both are wrong.

THE MORAL WEIGHT OF THE CONCLUSION

Criminal responsibility assessments carry moral weight because they influence how the system responds.

A finding that illness played a major role may open pathways to treatment-oriented legal outcomes. A finding that illness did not significantly shape the act may keep the case in a conventional criminal trajectory. Either way, the person remains human, the victim remains harmed, and the community remains small enough that everyone will live with the outcome.

As a visiting forensic psychiatrist, I felt that weight most sharply because I would eventually leave. My report would stay. My words would be read in court, debated by counsel, cited in decisions, remembered by families, and sometimes repeated in a community where stories travel faster than airplanes.

So I learned to write and speak with deliberate humility:

- To name uncertainty where it exists.
- To distinguish facts from inferences.
- To avoid theatrical certainty.
- To situate symptoms within chronology.
- To acknowledge context without collapsing into it.
- To keep the person's dignity intact even when describing harmful acts.

The Arctic taught me that criminal responsibility is not simply a determination about a moment in time. It is also a mirror held up to the system: how well it can see illness, how well it can see context, and how responsibly it can respond to both without turning either into an excuse or a weapon.

In the end, the question is not only what happened. It is also: what kind of justice, and what kind of care, are we capable of offering in a place where distance shapes everything?

CHAPTER 16

Risk Assessment in Small Communities

In the South, risk assessment often assumes distance. Distance between the accused and the complainant. Distance between a clinician and a community. Distance between what happens in court and what happens at the grocery store. Distance that allows anonymity to do some of the work, buffering contact, reducing friction, and making it plausible that no contact actually means no contact.

In the Arctic, distance is not the buffer. Connection is the reality.

Everyone is connected in ways that do not appear on a file: by kinship, by history, by proximity, by shared spaces, and by the simple fact that there may be one store, one school, one clinic, one road that everyone uses.

So when you sit down to assess violence risk, self-harm risk, and return-to-community realities, you quickly realize that the usual templates—neat, universal, portable—do not fit well here. You can still use structured thinking, but you have to translate it into a place where anonymity is impossible and where risk is rarely confined to one person's psychology.

It is social. It is logistical. It is relational. It is immediate.

EVERYONE IS CONNECTED

In a small northern community, the accused and the victim may be related, or may have children together, or may share extended family networks that cannot be untangled by a court order. The interpreter may know both parties.

The court worker may have gone to school with them. A nurse may be the cousin of someone in the case. A corrections officer may be a neighbor.

This does not mean professionals are incapable of professionalism. They are often exceptionally professional. But it does mean every interaction carries an added layer: people are not strangers to one another here.

That reality changes everything. It changes how much a victim can feel protected. It changes how willing an accused person is to speak openly. It changes how confidentiality works in practice, because even if no one says a word, presence alone communicates information: seeing someone enter a building, seeing a taxi stop, seeing a person sit in a waiting area.

It also changes risk management in the most basic way: the environment is small enough that people will run into each other. "Just avoid them" is not a plan.

SAFETY PLANNING WHEN ANONYMITY IS IMPOSSIBLE

In urban settings, safety planning often leans on services: shelters, alternative housing, supervised visitation, specialized programs, rapid police response, multiple clinics, multiple pharmacies, multiple places to go.

In the Arctic, the question is often painfully practical: where, exactly, can a person go that is safe and sustainable tonight?

Safety planning becomes a kind of engineering:

- Is there a safe house?
- Is there a family member who can host without creating new conflict?

- Is housing overcrowded?
- Can the person realistically comply with a curfew in that household?
- Can the victim realistically avoid the accused in a community where paths cross?
- If alcohol is a trigger, what does avoid alcohol mean in a place where people drink in private homes and everyone knows where it is happening?
- If the plan requires counselling, when is counselling available and how will attendance happen if weather cancels travel?

The best safety plans in small communities are not the most punitive. They are the most realistic. They acknowledge friction instead of pretending it will not happen. They build in early warning and rapid de-escalation, because preventing the next incident often depends on what happens in the first ten minutes of rising heat.

They are collaborative, because no single professional can manage risk alone in a place where relationships carry more weight than paperwork.

VIOLENCE RISK: BEYOND THE CHECKLIST

Structured professional judgment still matters. Patterns still matter. History still matters. But in the Arctic, violence risk is often inseparable from:

- Overcrowding and lack of private space
- Unresolved grief and trauma
- Substance use as coping and as social currency
- Repeated breaches that escalate despair and resentment
- Shame in small communities where reputation travels

- Intimate partner dynamics where separation is logistically difficult
- Limited access to ongoing therapy, anger work, and addictions care

This means risk can spike not only because a person is dangerous, but because conditions are combustible.

I learned to ask questions that sound less like a form and more like lived reality:

- When you get angry, what happens in your body first?
- What do you do when you feel disrespected?
- Where do you go to cool down?
- Who can you call that actually helps?
- What happens when you drink?
- What conditions have you breached before, and why?
- What would make you lose control again?

I also learned to treat protective factors with the same realism. A protective factor is not family support if the home is chaotic and violent. A protective factor is not employment if the job is seasonal and insecure. A protective factor is not community if the community is also the source of conflict. Protective factors have to be functional, not symbolic.

SELF-HARM RISK: THE QUIETEST EMERGENCY

Self-harm risk in custody is often visible: behavior changes, hopelessness, despair amplified by confinement.

Self-harm risk on return to the community can be quieter and, in some ways, more dangerous. A person is released into the same conditions that preceded the arrest: overcrowding, conflict, substance availability, shame, unresolved trauma, and limited follow-up. Sometimes what rises after release is not relief but collapse.

I learned to pay attention to transitional moments:

- The first 24 to 72 hours after release
- The first time the person runs into someone involved in the case
- The first time alcohol appears
- The first argument at home
- The first missed appointment
- The first night of insomnia

Self-harm risk is not always about wanting to die. Sometimes it is about wanting the pain to stop. Sometimes it is about shame. Sometimes it is about fear of retaliation. Sometimes it is about the crushing realization that the legal problem has ended but life has not improved.

In small communities, where privacy is thin, suicidal thinking can also be hidden behind performance: people keep their face intact until they can no longer maintain it.

So the safety plan has to be concrete:

- Who will check in, and how often?
- Where can the person go if they feel unsafe, physically or mentally?
- Is there an agreed exit plan from conflict (walk away, go to a specific house, call a specific person)?
- Are there means-safety steps that actually make sense in that household?
- Is there a plan for sleep, withdrawal, and cravings?

- Is there rapid access to the nursing station or crisis line that will actually answer?

A safety plan that cannot be executed in real time is not safety planning. It is documentation.

RETURN-TO-COMMUNITY REALITIES

Return to community is not a moment. It is a collision.

The person returns not only to a place, but to a network: family expectations, unresolved disputes, old loyalties, old grudges, social media, gossip, and the unavoidable visibility of being the person who was in court.

This is where the intimacy of public systems becomes clinically relevant. In the Arctic, a court decision echoes quickly. People know who was released. People know who has conditions. People know who is supposed to avoid whom.

That visibility can increase risk.

- A victim may feel unsafe even if conditions exist.
- An accused person may feel watched and humiliated.
- Families may feel divided.
- Old conflicts may reignite.

So return-to-community planning has to include the social layer:

- How will the person handle provocation?
- What will they do when someone brings up the case?
- Who can intervene before the situation escalates?
- What does stay away mean in a town where you will see each other?

- Can there be agreed routes and times that reduce accidental contact?
- Can there be structured supports that reduce boredom and relapse?

Sometimes, the most protective intervention is not a restriction but a structured day, something that reduces idle time, reduces exposure to triggers, and gives the nervous system a chance to settle.

THE ETHICAL TENSION: RISK LANGUAGE IN A CONNECTED WORLD

Writing about risk in a small community carries an ethical tension that I felt every time I drafted a report.

In a city, your words may disappear into a system. In the Arctic, your words can become part of someone's reputation.

Describing someone as high risk may be clinically justified, but it can also follow them in a place where people remember. Describing someone as low risk may feel reassuring, but it can also minimize a victim's fear in a community where fear has long memory.

So I learned to write and speak in a way that was specific rather than global:

- Not dangerous person, but risk increases under these conditions.
- Not safe, but risk appears lower when these supports are in place.
- Not noncompliant, but conditions have been breached when they were unrealistic or when substance use escalated.

Specificity is both clinically better and ethically safer.

WHAT THE ARCTIC TAUGHT ME ABOUT RISK

Risk assessment on circuit taught mc that risk is never only inside the person.

It lives in:

- A crowded house
- A cancelled flight
- An unanswered phone
- An impossible bail condition
- A community where everyone knows
- A history that cannot be outrun
- The fragile moments when someone is released back into it all

In small communities, the goal is not to eliminate risk. That is fantasy. The goal is to reduce predictable sparks, strengthen real protective factors, and build safety plans that survive the reality of weather, scarcity, and connection.

Because in the Arctic, anonymity will not protect anyone. Only realism will.

CHAPTER 17

Sentencing Reports and Moral Weight

A sentencing report is a strange document.

It is clinical writing aimed at a legal reader, composed in the shadow of harm, and destined to become part of a permanent record. It is written about a person at one of the worst points in their life, sometimes after an offence they regret, sometimes after an offence they deny, sometimes after an offence that has fractured a family or a community.

It is written with the knowledge that your words may shape what happens next: custody or community, treatment or punishment, conditions that support change or conditions that set someone up to fail. That is the moral weight of the report.

In the Arctic, the weight feels heavier, not because the law is different, but because everything is closer. The judge will not just sentence a name on paper. The judge will sentence someone whose family may be in the room, someone who may be related to the complainant, someone whose story will echo through a small place where no one disappears into a crowd. The system is public and intimate at the same time.

So when I sat down to write, I felt the tension immediately. I must be fair. I must be clear. I must not sentimentalize. I must not flatten.

MITIGATION, RESPONSIBILITY, REHABILITATION POTENTIAL

Sentencing reports often ask for three things, whether explicitly or implicitly:

1. **Mitigation:** What factors help explain how this person got here without excusing the harm?
2. **Responsibility:** What does accountability look like in this case, including recognition of harm and willingness to change?
3. **Rehabilitation potential:** What is realistically possible, given the person and the environment they will return to?

In southern settings, mitigation can sometimes be written as a list: childhood trauma, mental illness, substance use, poverty, loss. The list can become formulaic.

In the Arctic, mitigation has to be written with care, because context is not just background. It is often the main current that has carried the person into court.

Overcrowded housing. Food insecurity. Repeated exposure to violence. Early school disruption. Intergenerational trauma. Limited access to mental health care. Scarce addictions treatment. Geographic isolation.

None of these erase responsibility. But they shape what responsibility can reasonably look like.

It is easy to demand change as if people have the same range of options everywhere. It is harder, and more honest, to ask: What supports actually exist? What barriers will remain? What would success look like here, not in an ideal city?

Rehabilitation potential is not a moral judgment. It is a practical one. Practical judgments require knowledge of local reality.

WRITING FOR A JUDGE WHILE HONORING A PERSON'S STORY

Sentencing reports are read by judges who are under pressure: heavy dockets, limited time, competing narratives from Crown and defense, and the duty to keep the public safe while maintaining proportionality and fairness.

A judge does not need a novel. A judge needs clarity.

But a person is not a summary.

So the craft becomes finding the narrow space where both can be true: writing with the precision the court requires while refusing to erase the person's humanity.

I learned to structure reports in a way that respects the reader's needs without turning the subject into an object:

- What I was asked to do and what I did (sources, limitations, interpreter use)
- Clinical history that is relevant, not voyeuristic
- Mental state and diagnostic impressions, carefully grounded
- Risk formulation that is specific, not global
- Protective factors that are functional, not symbolic
- Mitigating factors framed as explanations, not excuses
- Treatment and rehabilitation recommendations that are realistic in the North
- A plain-language summary that makes the core points usable

Within that structure, I tried to keep one ethical commitment: never write about a person as if they are not going to read it. Even when they never do, that commitment protects tone. It keeps you from cruelty disguised as objectivity. It prevents the subtle dehumanization that can creep in when you write about offenders instead of people.

Honoring a person's story does not mean minimizing the harm they caused. It means holding the full picture:

- The harm done to the victim
- The choices made by the accused
- The vulnerabilities that shaped those choices
- The system conditions that intensified them
- The realistic pathways to reduce future harm

The story is not a justification. It is a map.

And the judge, ultimately, is being asked to decide what to do with that map.

MITIGATION WITHOUT ROMANCE

The Arctic can invite romantic narratives: resilience, vast landscapes, cultural richness. Those things are real. But forensic writing must resist romance, because romance can distort.

Mitigation is not poetry. It is specificity.

If trauma is relevant, explain how it relates to emotion regulation, threat perception, substance use, or impulsivity.

If cognitive limitations are relevant, describe how they affect learning from consequences, comprehension of conditions, and susceptibility to influence.

If substance use is relevant, differentiate between acute intoxication, substance use disorder severity, withdrawal risks, relapse triggers, and treatment history.

If grief is relevant, locate it in time and show how it changed function, mood, and coping.

The judge needs to understand mechanisms, not just adjectives. The person deserves to be understood as more than a label.

RESPONSIBILITY: THE HARDEST PARAGRAPH TO WRITE

Responsibility is often the hardest part, because it is ethically loaded.

Some people express remorse clearly. Some cannot. Some deny. Some are too ashamed to speak. Some are emotionally flattened by trauma or depression. Some are defensive because the legal process is adversarial.

The absence of visible remorse is not always the absence of responsibility, but it can also be a risk marker, depending on the context.

So I learned to write about responsibility in behavioral terms rather than moral tone:

- Did the person acknowledge the act?
- Did they acknowledge the impact on the victim?
- Did they show willingness to comply with supports?
- Did they engage with treatment in the past?

- What has happened after prior releases?
- What does their behavior suggest about insight and capacity for change?

Responsibility is not a feeling. It is an action path.

In the North, where follow-up can be fragile, an action path matters more than eloquent statements.

THE QUIET INFLUENCE OF A WELL-CRAFTED REPORT

Sentencing reports rarely make headlines. They do not feel dramatic in the moment. But their influence can be profound.

A careful report can:

- Prevent a court from imposing conditions that are impossible
- Reduce the cycle of breaches by recommending realistic structures
- Shift a judge's understanding from "bad person" to "person with predictable risk triggers"
- Highlight treatment needs that custody staff already see but cannot formalize
- Support a victim's safety by identifying specific risk conditions and prevention strategies
- Create a record that follows the person into future decisions, sometimes helping them, sometimes constraining them

The influence is quiet because it happens in the language of the system: paragraphs, formulations, recommendations. But in small communities, the ripple is not quiet at all. It shows up in whether someone stabilizes or spirals, whether a family holds together or fractures further, whether future harm is prevented or repeated.

This is why the moral weight matters.

In forensic work, it is tempting to protect yourself from weight by becoming technical, hiding behind jargon, behind diagnostic labels, behind neutral tone that is actually emotional distancing.

But in the Arctic, the closeness makes that harder. You see the people again. You see the same families. You see the same court workers, the same nurses, the same officers. You realize that your report is not a private academic exercise.

It is a piece of a community's story.

So I tried to write with a discipline that was both clinical and human:

- Grounded in facts
- Explicit about limitations
- Honest about uncertainty
- Careful with language that could stigmatize
- Specific about risk and protective factors
- Realistic about what rehabilitation can look like when geography sets the rules

A sentencing report is, at its best, a bridge between the law's need for clarity and a human life's need to be seen accurately.

That bridge carries moral weight because people walk on it:

- Victims
- Accused persons

- Families
- Communities

And if you build it poorly, someone falls.

CHAPTER 18

Treatment Orders, Diversion, and Therapeutic Jurisprudence

On circuit, you learn quickly that the justice system is asked to do too much.

It is asked to manage addiction, untreated psychosis, trauma, family violence, poverty, and housing collapse, often with tools designed mainly for one thing: adjudicating charges. When those tools do not fit the human problems arriving at the courthouse door, the system improvises. Sometimes it improvises harshly. Sometimes it improvises creatively.

That creativity is where you begin to hear words like diversion, treatment orders, and therapeutic jurisprudence, the idea that legal processes can be structured to support health, rehabilitation, and reduced harm, not only punishment.

In the Arctic, these concepts are both promising and frustrating because the law can gesture toward treatment even when treatment is not reliably available.

WHAT DIVERSION CAN, AND CANNOT, SOLVE

Diversion is often spoken of with hope, as if it is a switch that turns a legal problem into a health problem and then resolves it through care.

But diversion is not a cure. It is a pathway.

At its best, diversion can do several important things:

- Interrupt a cycle, keeping a person from accumulating convictions for behavior driven by untreated illness or addiction
- Reduce remand harm, avoiding the deterioration that comes from holding vulnerable people in custody
- Create leverage for engagement, sometimes the only reason someone accepts help is that the court creates a structured expectation
- Shift the narrative, reframing "noncompliance" and "bad choices" as treatable patterns with identifiable triggers
- Increase safety, when it leads to stabilization, reduced substance use, and stronger supports, it can reduce future harm to victims and the community

But diversion also has limits that become stark in the North.

Diversion cannot solve:

- Housing scarcity
- Food insecurity
- Overcrowding and family conflict
- Limited local clinical workforce
- Weather-related disruptions to appointments and travel
- The absence of detox beds, residential programs, or consistent outpatient services
- The reality that "treatment" may be a visiting team once a month

If diversion is used as a label without infrastructure, it becomes performative: a well-intentioned legal gesture that cannot be sustained. When it fails, the person is often blamed as if the failure were purely motivational.

This is one of the hardest truths I encountered: diversion can become a trap if it demands engagement in services that do not exist, or compliance with conditions that no one can realistically support.

Diversion is not a moral reward. It is a practical strategy. If the strategy has no supply line, it will collapse.

TREATMENT ORDERS: MEDICINE WITH LEGAL GRAVITY

Treatment orders, whether framed as conditions, mandated treatment participation, or other legal mechanisms, bring a special gravity. They turn "recommendation" into "requirement." They can feel coercive to the person. They can feel reassuring to the court. They can feel like a compromise between custody and release.

They also raise ethical questions that are sharper in remote settings:

- Is treatment being ordered because it is genuinely available, or because the court wishes it were available?
- Is the order likely to increase engagement, or likely to create breaches when services are interrupted?
- Will the person have the supports needed to comply (transport, phone access, stable housing, interpreter access)?
- Is the order proportionate to the offence and to the person's capacity?

A treatment order can stabilize a life if it is paired with real access.

But if the system cannot deliver access, the order can become a new kind of punishment: you must do the thing, the thing is not possible, you fail, you are breached, you return to custody.

That is the geography trap wearing a therapeutic mask.

COORDINATING WITH SCARCE COMMUNITY SUPPORTS

In the Arctic, the most important part of diversion and treatment orders is rarely the legal wording.

It is the coordination.

Coordination is the quiet labor that makes or breaks the plan. It is often carried by a small number of people who are already overextended: nurses at the health center, community mental health workers, court workers, probation officers, victim services staff, and sometimes Elders or community leaders who hold informal authority and trust.

As a visiting forensic psychiatrist, my recommendations were only as useful as their fit with this reality. Over time, I learned to ask questions that were not "clinical" in the traditional sense but were essential:

- Who is the point person in the community for follow-up?
- How often can the person realistically be seen?
- Is there a reliable phone? Is there privacy to use it?
- If the plan relies on telehealth, where will the session occur?
- What happens when weather cancels travel?
- What supports exist for substance use, formal or informal?
- Are there culturally grounded resources the person trusts?

- What do we do after hours, when crises often peak?

Coordination in the North is less about building a perfect plan and more about building a plan that survives disruption.

That means contingency thinking:

- If counselling is cancelled, what is the backup?
- If medication runs out, who can bridge it?
- If the person relapses, what is the response that reduces harm instead of escalating to breach immediately?
- If conflict rises at home, where can the person go safely for a cooling-off period?

This kind of planning is not glamorous, but it is therapeutic jurisprudence in its most honest form: law structured around the real conditions of life.

THERAPEUTIC JURISPRUDENCE: HOPEFUL, BUT NOT NAÏVE

Therapeutic jurisprudence can sound soft to people who have seen violence and are tired of systems making excuses. But in practice, it is not softness. It is realism.

It is the recognition that punishment alone does not treat psychosis, does not treat addiction, does not heal trauma, and does not create housing.

It is also the recognition that victims deserve safety that actually holds, not safety written on paper.

In the Arctic, therapeutic jurisprudence is meaningful when it does three things:

1. Targets the drivers of risk, including symptoms, addiction, impulsivity, and trauma triggers.
2. Uses conditions sparingly and realistically, so compliance is possible and meaningful.
3. Builds genuine continuity, so the plan can continue after court day ends.

When those elements are present, diversion can be powerful. It can reduce the churn of remand. It can reduce breach cycles. It can help a person stabilize enough to begin real change.

When those elements are absent, diversion becomes a label the system uses to feel progressive, while the person continues to cycle through the same outcomes.

WHAT STAYED WITH ME

What stayed with me most was how often the success of diversion depended less on the person's motivation and more on whether the system could meet them halfway.

In the South, halfway is usually nearby.

In the Arctic, halfway can be a plane ride away.

So the ethical task for a visiting forensic psychiatrist is to recommend diversion and treatment orders with disciplined realism, anchored in what exists, explicit about what does not, and careful not to turn scarcity into blame.

Because diversion can open a door.

But a door that opens onto an empty hallway is not a solution.

It is just another kind of waiting.

PART V

THE HOTEL BETWEEN WORLDS

CHAPTER 19

Evenings: Notes, Calls, and the Knock on the Door

In the South, the end of the workday usually has edges.

You leave the hospital. You step into your car. You cross an invisible boundary between professional life and personal time. Even if you carry work home in your head, the world around you changes. The walls change. The sounds change. The air changes.

On circuit, evenings do not have edges.

Evenings are where the day folds inward, court, jail, nursing station, into a single quiet room with a desk, a lamp, and a stack of unfinished sentences that must become a report by morning.

The hotel becomes the clinic.

The hotel becomes the office.

Sometimes the hotel becomes the on-call unit.

And you become, once again, the visitor who has to make the time hold.

WRITING REPORTS LATE

By the time I returned to the hotel after a day of interviews and court appearances, my body would feel both heavy and alert, fatigued from cold and movement but wired by the intensity of what I had just heard. The mind resists sleep when it has been holding other people's stories too tightly.

I would sit at the desk, open my notebook, and begin the second shift.

The writing is not just transcription. It is translation.

You translate a person's spoken account into something legible for the court. You translate symptoms into diagnostic language. You translate uncertainty into probabilities without pretending it is certainty. You translate context into mitigation without romanticizing. You translate risk into recommendations without turning a person into a danger label.

And you do all of it while knowing that you may have only hours before the next court day begins.

A northern hotel room is not designed for careful forensic writing. The chair is slightly wrong. The light is too harsh or too dim. The desk is too small. The walls are too thin. The hallway outside carries voices. The heater clicks. The window holds darkness.

But the report has to be written anyway, because tomorrow the circuit moves. The system does not pause for your fatigue.

I learned to write in the way you travel in the North: efficiently, deliberately, always aware that a disruption could arrive without warning.

ANSWERING URGENT CONSULTS

And then there were the calls.

A nurse from the health center needing a quick opinion about a patient whose mood had collapsed after court.

A corrections officer asking whether a presentation looked like withdrawal or psychosis.

A court worker checking whether an assessment could happen earlier than planned because an unexpected docket change had opened a window.

A lawyer asking for clarification, what I meant by a phrase, whether a conclusion could be stated more plainly, whether a particular recommendation was realistic.

Sometimes the calls were routine.

Sometimes they were not.

Sometimes they carried the quiet urgency that makes you sit up straighter before you even know why: someone is escalating, someone is refusing, someone is self-harming, someone is hearing voices, someone is being held in segregation and the staff are worried.

On circuit, you can be asked to be many things quickly. Advisor. Consultant. Interpreter of symptoms. Translator for legal readers. Risk assessor. Sometimes, uncomfortably, arbiter of what the system should do next when there are no good options.

And because resources are thin, the question behind the call is often unspoken but clear:

If you do not help us decide, who will?

That question turns your hotel room into an on-call unit, even when you technically are not "on call."

Because in a place where specialists visit, the presence of a specialist is treated as a resource not to be wasted.

THE HOTEL AS AN "ON-CALL UNIT"

Over time, I stopped thinking of the hotel as accommodation and began thinking of it as a staging area.

The lobby was a waiting room in disguise.

The hallway was a corridor where confidentiality was fragile.

The restaurant was a place where you might see a lawyer, a court worker, a nurse, a corrections officer, a patient's family member, all within the same ten minutes.

Even the elevator could become a clinical space, not because you wanted it to, but because small communities do not separate roles neatly.

Someone might stop you casually: "Doctor, can I ask you something?"

Someone might lower their voice: "He's not doing well."

Someone might simply look at you with the kind of eyes that ask for help without using words.

It is hard to explain to people who have never done circuit work how a hotel can become part of the clinical system. But it does. Not formally, not on paper, but informally and inevitably. It becomes the place where you write, think, consult, and sometimes receive urgent information when there is nowhere else to put it.

The hotel holds the work the way the tundra holds tracks: quietly, without commentary, but unmistakably.

THE KNOCK ON THE DOOR

The knock is what makes it real.

Not every trip had one, but when it happened, it reset the nervous system instantly.

A knock late in the evening carries a particular meaning when you are in a distant place on a forensic circuit. It is rarely social. It is rarely casual. It is usually either:

- a request for immediate help, or
- an unexpected complication, or

- a boundary moment you have to navigate carefully.

Sometimes it was hotel staff delivering something banal, a key issue, a message.

But sometimes it was a professional colleague, court staff, nursing, or corrections standing in the hallway with urgency contained in a quiet face.

Those moments pull you out of writing and back into the system instantly. Your mind shifts gears in a second. The report sentence remains unfinished on the page, but your role changes.

And role-switching is one of the hidden stressors of circuit work.

EMOTIONAL WHIPLASH: CLINICIAN → EXPERT → WITNESS

In one day, sometimes in one hour, you might move through three identities:

1. **Clinician**—In the interview room, you are trying to listen deeply. You are trying to see the person as more than the offence. You are asking about trauma, grief, psychosis, withdrawal, suicidal thoughts. You are holding pain carefully, offering dignity in a place where dignity is often scarce.

2. **Expert**—Then you step into court, and the language changes. You become precise. You become structured. You translate your observations into legal relevance. You choose words that will stand up under scrutiny. You say less, not more, because your words carry weight.

3. **Witness**—And sometimes you become something else again: a witness in the moral sense. Someone who has seen enough to understand how fragile the system is, how heavy the stories are, how

thin the supports can be, and how much of the outcome depends on the luck of weather, timing, and staffing.

That last role is rarely acknowledged, but it is the one that follows you into the hotel room at night.

It is what makes it hard to sleep even when you are exhausted.

Because witnessing is not an action you can turn off by closing your laptop.

THE NIGHT WORK

Late in the evening, after the last call, after the last paragraph, I would sometimes sit back and feel the strange contradiction of circuit work:

- You are intensely involved in people's lives, and yet you are temporary.
- You are asked to provide clarity, and yet you are working with fragments.
- You are expected to be composed, and yet you carry stories that would unsettle anyone.

The hotel room holds all of that. It holds the unfinished drafts and the ethical tension. It holds the fatigue and the adrenaline. It holds the knowledge that tomorrow will begin early and the docket will not care how late you wrote.

And still, you write.

Because the report is not just paperwork. In places where resources are scarce and options are few, a well-formed report can shape decisions that keep someone safer, guide a judge toward realism, and sometimes, quietly, give a person a chance to be seen accurately rather than reduced to a label.

So you answer the calls.

You keep the phone close.

You listen for the knock.

And you learn to switch roles without losing yourself, because in the Arctic, the work does not stay neatly inside the building where it began.

CHAPTER 20

Confidentiality in a Small Place

In the South, confidentiality often feels like architecture. Doors that close. Separate waiting rooms. Private offices. The anonymity of crowds. The comfortable assumption that if you do not tell anyone, no one will know.

In the Arctic, confidentiality is not architecture.

It is behavior.

It is a practice you perform in public spaces, repeatedly, with discipline, because the environment does not give you privacy by default. Small places do not have enough distance for secrecy to happen on its own.

And on circuit, you quickly learn that confidentiality is not only about what you say.

It is also about what your presence reveals.

SEEING PATIENTS IN HALLWAYS, STORES, LOBBIES

It happens sooner than you expect.

You finish an interview in the jail and return to the hotel. You step into the lobby and see someone you assessed earlier, now with family, or with a court worker, or alone near the front desk.

You go to the restaurant and recognize a face in the corner booth.

You walk into a store to buy water or snacks and realize the person standing near the aisle is the complainant in a case, or the accused person's cousin, or someone whose name is in your notes.

Sometimes it is the patient who sees you first. Sometimes it is you.

And in that split second, you have to decide how to move your body, where to place your eyes, whether to nod, whether to pretend you did not see them, whether a neutral greeting would expose them, whether the absence of greeting would feel like rejection.

There are no perfect answers, only careful ones.

In urban practice, you can usually avoid these encounters. In the Arctic, you cannot. The same hotels, the same taxis, the same stores, the same corridors hold everyone: court staff, lawyers, nurses, guards, families, accused persons, victims, interpreters.

The system is public, and your work is stitched into it.

So confidentiality becomes a daily discipline of small decisions:

- Do I acknowledge?
- Do I wait for them to acknowledge?
- Do I move away?
- Do I keep my face neutral?
- Do I risk looking cold?
- Do I risk looking familiar?

What looks like a social gesture in the South can become a breach of privacy in the North.

BOUNDARIES: WHERE PROFESSIONALISM BECOMES VISIBLE

Boundaries in forensic psychiatry are always important. But in small communities, boundaries are not just ethical, they are protective.

They protect patients from exposure.

They protect victims from perceived partiality.

They protect local staff from gossip that can harm their credibility.

And they protect the visitor, because when you are temporary, misunderstandings can be amplified.

A casual conversation can be misread as favoritism.

A friendly greeting can be interpreted as alliance.

A shared taxi ride can become a rumor.

The community is small enough that stories travel faster than explanations.

So you learn to be warm without being familiar.

You learn to be respectful without being close.

You learn to show human decency while keeping a professional distance that is not personal.

This is harder than it sounds because the Arctic has a social closeness that can feel welcoming. People speak to each other. People help each other. People notice when you are new. If you are not careful, you can drift into social intimacy without intending to.

But forensic work requires neutrality, not emotional neutrality, but role neutrality. You can be compassionate and still not be aligned.

And in a small place, neutrality is tested constantly.

DUAL RELATIONSHIPS: THE INEVITABILITY YOU MUST MANAGE

In big cities, dual relationships are often preventable. You can refer out. You can transfer care. You can avoid social overlap.

In the Arctic, overlap is built into the environment.

The interpreter may be related to the person you are assessing.

The nurse may be the neighbor of the complainant.

The court worker may have grown up with the accused.

The corrections officer may be dating someone in the extended family network.

Even you, as a visitor, can become part of the overlap simply by staying in the same hotel as everyone else.

Dual relationships here are not always ethical violations. Often they are simply a reality of community life. The ethical question becomes:

How do we manage overlap without pretending it does not exist?

That means being explicit with interpreters about confidentiality. It means checking whether someone feels comfortable. It means being prepared to adjust if a conflict is identified. It means documenting carefully when needed. It means understanding that privacy looks different in communities where relational networks are dense.

It also means refusing to exploit familiarity. Just because someone "knows the family" does not mean their knowledge is yours to use casually. Community knowledge is not a free resource. It belongs to the people who hold it, and it has consequences if mishandled.

RESPECTFUL DISTANCE: THE ETHICS OF HOW YOU MOVE

Over time, I developed a way of moving through public spaces that felt like a northern form of professionalism.

In lobbies and hallways, I avoided initiating greetings with people I had assessed, unless they greeted me first. If they did greet me, I responded briefly and neutrally, polite, human, not cold, but without anything that would suggest familiarity.

In stores, if I recognized someone, I did not approach. I did not engage. I did not check in. Even if the clinician in me wanted to ask how they were doing, the forensic professional in me knew the cost of that impulse. The person might be with family. The person might be with someone who does not know they were in custody. The person might not want their connection to the system exposed.

Sometimes respectful distance feels like indifference. It is not.

It is protection.

I also learned to manage my own visibility. In small communities, the visitor is noticeable. Where you sit, where you eat, who you talk to, it all becomes data in the social world.

So I was careful. Not paranoid, but aware.

Because confidentiality is not only about the patient. It is also about the integrity of the system. Victims deserve to trust that the professional involved is not casually socializing with the accused. Accused persons deserve to trust that they will not be exposed. Court staff deserve to trust that their work will not be complicated by rumors of improper closeness.

In the Arctic, trust is not built through grand gestures. It is built through repeated small acts of restraint.

THE EMOTIONAL COST OF RESTRAINT

There is an emotional cost to maintaining boundaries in a small place.

As a visitor, you can feel lonely. You may want to be friendly. You may want to connect. You may feel the instinct to soften the formality because the environment feels human and close.

But you also carry stories that are heavy, and the instinct to seek comfort through social warmth can be strong, especially after difficult interviews.

The discipline is to find your support in appropriate places: professional colleagues who understand, private reflection, scheduled debriefs, calls home, writing. Not in the accidental intimacy of a lobby conversation with someone whose life is entangled in the cases you are working on.

This is not just self-protection. It is ethical practice.

CONFIDENTIALITY AS A NORTHERN SKILL

In the end, confidentiality in a small place is not something you "have." It is something you do.

You do it when you meet someone's eyes and choose not to signal recognition.

You do it when you keep your voice even and your words minimal.

You do it when you resist the urge to ask questions in public.

You do it when you treat every hallway as potentially public, every lobby as potentially observed, every casual moment as part of a wider social web.

And you do it with humility, because you will never control the community's knowledge completely. People will still talk. People will still infer. Privacy will still be imperfect.

But you can ensure that you do not become the leak.

That is what respectful distance means in the Arctic: not coldness, not superiority, not detachment, but carefulness.

A quiet form of care.

In a place where everyone sees everyone, confidentiality is not a rule written in policy.

It is a posture you carry wherever you go.

CHAPTER 21

The Social Worker, the Court Worker, the Escort

If you wanted to understand how the northern justice-and-care system actually worked, you did not start with the judge.

You started with the people who moved everything.

The social worker who knew which family was hanging on by a thread.

The court worker who could explain a court order in plain language without humiliating anyone.

The escort who could get someone from the jail to court and back again safely, calmly, and without turning the transfer into another trauma.

They were not the loudest people in the system, but they were the ones who made the system possible. Their work was not ornamental. It was structural.

On circuit, I learned to watch them the way you watch the weather, because everything depended on their steadiness.

UNSUNG LABOR

There is a kind of labor that never gets named in reports.

Not because it is not important, but because it is so constant that it becomes invisible, until it fails, and then everyone realizes what it was holding.

TRANSPORT

Transport in the Arctic is not a minor logistical step. It is a daily negotiation with cold, distance, staffing, and timing.

The escort who brings someone to court is not simply walking them across a hallway. They are managing risk, dignity, and unpredictability. They are reading body language, anticipating escalation, adjusting tone, and keeping the person moving without provoking shame. They are doing this in a place where everyone might recognize the person being escorted.

Even the act of moving someone can expose them.

A transfer becomes a public event.

So escorts learn to move people with efficiency and minimal spectacle, because in small communities, spectacle has consequences.

TRANSLATION

Interpreters are not just translating vocabulary. They are translating meaning across worlds, often while carrying their own emotional load, often while navigating conflicts of interest that urban systems rarely force on people.

But the court worker and the social worker do a kind of translation too, translation of systems.

They translate legal language into something understandable.

They translate clinical recommendations into steps that might actually happen.

They translate conditions into daily routines.

They translate the system's demands into something that will not break the person immediately.

Sometimes they also translate the person back to the system, helping the court see that a breach was not simply defiance, that silence was not necessarily guilt, that confusion was not a performance.

They are translators of human complexity.

PAPERWORK

Paperwork sounds trivial until you realize that paperwork is how help becomes real.

Forms determine whether someone gets a travel voucher, whether a referral is accepted, whether a medication is renewed, whether a bed is arranged, whether a court date is confirmed, whether a treatment appointment is scheduled, whether a victim receives support.

In northern systems, paperwork is more than bureaucracy, it is a survival tool.

And the people who do it are often working with outdated computers, limited time, interrupted internet, long queues of urgent needs, and no guarantee that the plan will hold because a flight can cancel everything.

They do it anyway.

DE-ESCALATION

The most important work I saw was often the work no one noticed: the quiet, skilled de-escalation that prevented a crisis from becoming a violent incident or a self-harm attempt.

The social worker who knew not to push too hard when someone's shame was rising.

The court worker who could read a person's face in the courtroom and step in before panic became disruption.

The escort who could shift the tone, soften the voice, slow the pace, and offer a simple instruction so that a transfer did not become a struggle.

De-escalation is not a personality trait. It is a skill built through repetition, patience, and the painful knowledge of what happens when things go wrong.

It is also a form of care.

SHARED FATIGUE

Circuit work compresses time, and that compression produces fatigue that settles into the body.

You see it in the eyes first.

The social worker who has heard too many stories of harm and too few stories of repair.

The court worker who has explained the same conditions a hundred times and still watches people breach because the conditions do not fit the life.

The escort who has been on their feet all day, managing tension that could erupt without warning, and then has to go home and be a parent, a partner, a member of a small community that knows exactly what they do for work.

Fatigue in small systems is not just tiredness. It is exposure.

Exposure to trauma, conflict, suffering, and the limits of what can be done.

And there is a particular exhaustion that comes from being the person who is expected to hold things together when the infrastructure is thin. There are no extra staff waiting in the wings. There is no easy referral to a bigger program down the road. There is no anonymous specialist clinic where you can send the hardest cases.

Sometimes there is only you, doing the work again tomorrow.

As a visitor, I felt a different kind of fatigue, but theirs was heavier in one crucial way:

They could not leave.

They lived inside the system they served. They would see the same faces again at the store, at school events, at community gatherings. Their work followed them into their personal lives, because in the Arctic the boundary between professional world and community world is thin.

SHARED PURPOSE

And yet, what stayed with me was not only the fatigue.

It was the purpose.

Most people do not take on this kind of work by accident. They do it because they believe, quietly and stubbornly, that it matters.

Purpose shows up in small acts:

- A court worker taking extra time to explain a condition until the person can repeat it back.
- A social worker calling multiple numbers until they reach someone who can help.
- An escort moving with calm dignity even when the person is insulting them.
- An interpreter asking for clarification rather than smoothing over meaning, because accuracy matters.

- Someone staying late to complete paperwork so that a referral does not die in the gap.

Purpose also shows up in how they treat the visitor.

They orient you. They correct you gently. They warn you about what will not work. They help you avoid mistakes that would harm trust. They lend you their local knowledge without making you feel incompetent, because they want the work to go well, not because they want credit.

In those moments, you realize something important:

The system does not run on policies alone.

It runs on relationships and stamina.

THE QUIET PARTNERSHIP

As a forensic psychiatrist, my name went on the report. My opinions were quoted. My conclusions carried the sheen of expertise.

But the truth is that my work was scaffolded by people whose names often never appeared in the official record.

The social worker who gathered background information and made referrals.

The court worker who bridged culture, language, and law.

The escort who ensured safety without humiliation.

They were not just supports to my work. They were co-authors of the system's functioning, day after day.

And in a place where the margin for error is thin, their competence was not optional.

It was the difference between a day that held and a day that broke.

Circuit work can make you feel like the visitor is the main character.

But the longer you stay, the clearer it becomes:

The real story belongs to the people who stay behind after the plane takes off and return to the work the next morning, carrying shared fatigue and shared purpose into another day that has to be made possible.

PART VI

PEOPLE BEHIND FILES

CHAPTER 22

The Young Person With Too Many Breaches

He was young enough that the file felt heavier than it should have.

Not because it was thick, though it was, but because the dates inside it were too close together. Charges stacked like winter days when the light barely changes: breach, breach, breach, failure to comply, failure to appear, breach again. Reading it, you could almost feel the system losing patience in real time.

By the time I met him, noncompliance had become his unofficial diagnosis.

It followed him through the paperwork the way a shadow follows a person across snow. It showed up in the language of the record, does not listen, does not follow rules, does not show up, does not learn. It showed up in the tone of institutional fatigue, the resigned belief that this was simply who he was.

But when he sat down in front of me, what I saw first was not defiance.

It was restlessness.

His leg bounced. His hands moved. His eyes flicked toward the door, toward the corners, toward me, away again. He spoke quickly in bursts, then paused as if his mind had taken a different exit. He answered some questions with too much detail, then could not remember the simplest sequence of events. He agreed too quickly, then contradicted himself without noticing.

He looked older than his age in the face, and younger than his age in his emotional reach.

I had seen this pattern before, in different places, in different systems. The label changes, troublemaker, bad kid, impulsive, angry, oppositional, but the nervous system underneath is familiar.

A life spent surviving without enough structure.

A brain that runs hot, fast, and hungry.

ADHD, TRAUMA, SUBSTANCE USE, UNSTABLE HOUSING

The story, when it emerged, did not arrive in clean chapters.

It arrived in fragments.

School never really worked. Not because he was unintelligent, but because sitting still felt like being trapped, and concentration felt like trying to hold water in a fist. He was in trouble early, talking, moving, leaving his seat, not finishing assignments, losing things, forgetting instructions. The adults around him responded the way institutions often respond: repeated discipline without understanding.

Somewhere along the way, the child learned a lesson that looked like behavior but was actually injury:

If you are going to be punished anyway, you might as well stop trying to please them.

Then trauma entered, not as a single dramatic event, but as a climate. Conflict. Violence exposure. Adults whose moods were unpredictable. Nights where sleep was not safe. Loss that was never properly mourned. Shame that grew quietly.

His attention problems did not exist beside trauma; they braided with it. Hyperactivity turned into hypervigilance. Impulsivity turned into reactivity. Poor emotional regulation turned into quick fights, quick exits, quick decisions he regretted later.

And then substance use entered, as it so often does, not as a party, but as a tool.

A way to slow the mind down.

A way to sleep.

A way to stop thinking.

A way to belong.

A way to mute the constant internal noise that ADHD and trauma can create when untreated.

By the time the system began naming addiction, it was already woven into his coping. And by the time the system began naming trauma, it had already shaped his default response to stress: fight, flee, numb.

Housing was never stable. When you do not have stable housing, you do not have stable anything else. You do not have a consistent routine. You do not have a quiet place to sleep. You do not have a reliable way to keep documents safe. You do not have a reliable phone. You do not have a predictable way to get to appointments. You do not have a corner of the world that belongs to you.

So when the court wrote conditions like a checklist, curfew, abstain, attend, report, avoid, comply, the list did not land on a stable life.

It landed on chaos.

And chaos does what it always does: it breaks plans.

NONCOMPLIANCE REFRAMED AS CHAOS AND SCARCITY

The file described him as noncompliant.

But when we looked closely at the breaches, a different story appeared.

He missed probation because he did not have a working phone and did not know the office hours, and when he finally arrived it was late and he felt humiliated and left.

He breached a curfew because he did not have a safe place to stay and the house he was supposed to be in became volatile at night.

He failed to appear because he slept through the morning after three nights of insomnia and withdrawal and being moved around in custody, and no one had explained the date in a way he could retain.

He violated a no-contact order because no contact was impossible in a small place where people share stores, taxis, and family networks, and because he did not have the executive functioning to plan routes and avoidance strategies like a lawyer imagining the city.

He consumed alcohol because he was dependent and there was no consistent treatment support, and because abstinence was ordered like a moral demand instead of treated like a clinical pathway.

If you looked at those breaches with a purely moral lens, you could call them choices.

If you looked at them with a clinical lens, you could see patterns: executive dysfunction, poor working memory, impulsivity under stress, trauma-driven reactivity, addiction-driven craving, and the relentless pressure of scarcity.

The more accurate word was not noncompliance.

It was disorganization, not laziness, but a life without scaffolding.

It was dysregulation, not attitude, but a nervous system that had learned to run on emergency settings.

It was poverty of options, the quiet truth that many choices are made inside narrow corridors.

THE COURTROOM'S IMPATIENCE AND THE BRAIN'S REALITY

The justice system values consistency. It values compliance. It values predictable behavior.

ADHD, trauma, addiction, and unstable housing produce the opposite: inconsistency, missed steps, reactive decisions, and promises that are sincere in the moment but collapse under pressure.

This is where the young person with too many breaches becomes a permanent client of the system, not because they are destined for crime, but because the system's expectations are built for people with executive functioning and stability.

And when those are absent, the system interprets failure as defiance.

The tragedy is that the more the system punishes the failure, the more instability it creates:

- Remand disrupts routine further.
- Custody worsens sleep.
- Stigma worsens shame.
- Housing collapses while the person is held.
- Relationships fracture.

- Substance use rebounds on release.

And the next breach arrives like a scheduled event.

It becomes a self-fulfilling cycle. The system demands structure from a person whose life has none, and then punishes them for not producing it.

A DIFFERENT KIND OF QUESTION

When I sat with him, the most important question was not, "Why don't you comply?"

It was: "What would make compliance possible?"

Not in theory. In reality.

Could conditions be simplified, with fewer rules, clearer rules, rules that can be remembered?

Could supports be anchored, with one consistent contact person, one routine, one place to show up?

Could there be a plan for the first 72 hours after release: sleep, food, a phone, a check-in?

Could substance use expectations be paired with actual steps: harm reduction, withdrawal management, realistic treatment access?

Could the system recognize that punishment does not teach executive functioning?

Because executive functioning is not a moral skill. It is a brain-based skill.

And when that skill is impaired, by ADHD, by trauma, by addiction, by sleep deprivation, by chaos, people do not "learn" the way courts expect them to learn.

They repeat.

WHAT STAYED WITH ME

What stayed with me was how young he still was under all the breaches.

How quickly the file had aged him.

How the system had begun to treat him like a fixed problem, when he was still an unfinished person.

And how much of his so-called noncompliance made sense once you stopped reading it as willful failure and started reading it as the predictable outcome of a life lived without enough stability, without enough treatment, and without enough room to recover.

When I returned to my hotel that night to write, I felt the moral pressure of naming this accurately.

Because labels matter.

If you call it noncompliance, you justify tightening the net.

If you call it chaos and scarcity, you create the possibility of building a net that actually holds.

Not to excuse harm.

Not to minimize victim safety.

But to acknowledge a truth that is uncomfortable for systems:

Sometimes the person is not refusing the plan.

Sometimes the plan is refusing the person.

And the young person with too many breaches is the one who pays for that mismatch, again and again, until someone finally decides to treat the chaos, not just punish the fallout.

CHAPTER 23

The Man Everyone Fears, and No One Helped Early

By the time his name reached me, it had already arrived with a mood.

A tightening in the voice when people mentioned him. A pause in conversation, brief, practiced, familiar. A look that said, be careful, without having to use the words. In small communities, fear is not abstract. It has a tone. It has a posture. It has a memory.

"He's dangerous."

Sometimes people said it plainly. Sometimes they said it with euphemisms, "he can go off," "he's unpredictable," "he's got a temper." But the message was consistent. This was someone the system watched closely, someone staff prepared for, someone families avoided when they could, someone whose presence in a room changed the temperature.

And yet, when I read his history, what struck me first was not the violence.

It was the timeline.

Because the fear did not begin with the offence that brought him to court. The fear began years earlier, in small escalations that looked, at the time, like "behavior problems," "drinking," "trouble," "domestic conflict," "anger issues." The familiar early warning signs of a life moving toward collision.

No one helped early.

Or perhaps people tried in small ways, and the system could not hold it. Perhaps there were moments of concern that faded. Perhaps there were referrals that went nowhere. Perhaps there were missed appointments that became "noncompliance." Perhaps there were crises that were managed and then forgotten. In remote settings, "early intervention" often means that someone noticed, and then time passed.

By the time the file becomes thick, the window has narrowed.

By the time fear becomes a community fact, the options have shrunk.

ESCALATING VIOLENCE: A PATTERN, NOT A SURPRISE

His story was not one of sudden evil. It was one of repeated escalation.

The early incidents were often described as "minor": yelling, threats, property damage, punching walls, public intoxication, arguments that became physical. The kinds of incidents that a strained system can dismiss as routine, especially when they happen in the shadow of widespread substance use and normalized conflict.

But violence has a learning curve. If it works, if it creates distance, silence, compliance, fear, it reinforces itself.

Over time, the pattern hardened:

- Alcohol and conflict.
- Conflict and humiliation.
- Humiliation and rage.
- Rage and violence.
- Violence and short-term control.

Then remorse, or denial, or both. Then the cycle again.

In small communities, escalation is not contained. It is witnessed. People remember. Children absorb it. Partners adapt around it. Friends decide whether to intervene or stay away. The system responds episodically, often after something has already happened.

That episodic response can unintentionally train the person. Consequences arrive late, unpredictably, and then recede.

Which means the person never truly encounters a consistent boundary paired with consistent help.

SHAME AND LOSS: THE HIDDEN FUEL

What people saw was anger.

What I suspected, carefully and without romanticizing, was shame.

Shame is one of the most volatile emotions in forensic work. It is quiet until it is not. It lives under the surface, and then it erupts as rage when a person feels exposed, disrespected, powerless, or laughed at.

In his history, there were repeated losses: relationships ending, employment instability, family fracture, perhaps bereavement, perhaps the slow loss of social standing. In small communities, reputations are not private. When someone begins to be known as “dangerous,” they lose more than freedom. They lose belonging.

Some people respond to that with withdrawal.

Others respond with defiance.

And some respond with violence, not because violence is the true goal, but because violence is the only remaining tool for preserving a sense of power when everything else has eroded.

Shame can make a person double down. It can make apology impossible because apology feels like annihilation. It can make treatment feel like weakness. It can make any attempt to help feel like an insult.

If you do not recognize shame, you misread the person as purely antisocial.

And then you treat them as a pure threat.

Which can become self-fulfilling.

THE SYSTEM'S POSTURE: RISK MANAGEMENT

When someone becomes "the man everyone fears," systems move into a particular posture.

Containment.

Risk management becomes the dominant language. Staff focus on procedures: separation, restraints, segregation, security planning, conditions, no-contact orders, curfews, abstinence demands.

All necessary at times.

But risk management is not the same thing as change.

Risk management asks, how do we prevent the next incident?

Change asks, how does this person learn to live differently?

The first can be achieved through control.

The second cannot.

Control can stop behavior temporarily. It can create breathing room. It can protect victims and staff. But without an actual change pathway, treatment, consistent intervention, meaningful accountability, and supports that survive release, the behavior returns.

Often worse.

Because every cycle adds more shame, more loss, more resentment, and more hopelessness.

And hopelessness is dangerous in people who already externalize pain.

RISK MANAGEMENT VS ACTUAL CHANGE

This is where forensic psychiatry has to be honest.

There are cases where the immediate priority must be safety. Where risk is high. Where a person's violence is repeated, severe, and escalating. Where the community's fear is not prejudice but lived experience.

In those cases, you cannot write your way into a soft landing. You cannot recommend "anger management" as if it is a magic cure. You cannot pretend that a few sessions will undo decades of learning and harm.

But you also cannot stop at "dangerous."

If you stop at dangerous, you give the system only one option: hold, restrain, punish, isolate, and hope time changes what time rarely changes.

Actual change requires something more difficult:

- a coherent formulation that goes beyond "bad person"
- a recognition of substance use dynamics, if present
- a careful assessment of trauma and attachment history, without excusing harm
- an evaluation of personality structure and emotional regulation capacity
- targeted interventions that address shame, impulsivity, and threat perception

- consistent consequences paired with consistent support
- long-term follow-up that survives geography and staffing gaps
- and often, a culturally grounded approach that does not replicate the very power dynamics that fueled the person's mistrust

In the Arctic, the tragedy is that these resources are often thin or absent.

The system becomes very good at managing risk in the short term and very poor at enabling change in the long term.

So the man everyone fears becomes a chronic client of custody.

Not because he is destined to be, but because early help did not happen, and later help is harder, costlier, and more complex.

THE MORAL DISCOMFORT

There is a moral discomfort in seeing someone late.

It feels like being asked to assess a fire after it has already taken the house. People want to know why it happened. People want to know whether it will happen again. People want to know what to do now.

And you can answer those questions, partly.

But you also see the earlier moments, the smaller fires, that were never fully addressed. The opportunities where someone might have been diverted into treatment before the violence became identity, before fear became the community's default posture.

In remote systems, those opportunities are often lost not because people are indifferent, but because the infrastructure for early help is fragile: long waits, limited clinicians, high turnover, and the everyday demands of survival that push mental health down the list until it becomes crisis.

WHAT I WROTE, AND WHAT I CARRIED

When I returned to the hotel to write about him, I felt the tension that sits at the heart of forensic work:

- I must describe risk accurately, because safety is real.
- I must honor victims' fear, because harm has occurred.
- I must not minimize the pattern, because the pattern is the pattern.
- But I must also refuse to declare the person beyond help simply because help arrived late.

Because if we decide he is beyond help, we turn risk management into life management.

We accept permanent containment as the only answer.

And we ignore the hard lesson his story teaches:

Fear did not appear out of nowhere.

It was built over time, by escalating violence, by shame, by loss, and by the quiet absence of early intervention.

The man everyone fears is not just a person.

He is also a systems outcome.

And if the system wants fewer men like him, it cannot rely only on custody and conditions.

It has to build pathways for actual change, before fear becomes the only language left.

CHAPTER 24

The Woman on Remand Far From Her Children

She arrived in my schedule the way many women arrive in forensic systems: quietly.

Not high profile. Not dangerous. Not the kind of file that triggers a warning in the hallway. Her charges looked ordinary to the docket: an argument that went too far, a breach, a night where police were called, a situation that had already been deteriorating long before the system showed up to document it.

But when I met her, the first thing I noticed wasn't the charge.

It was the way her eyes kept returning to the same place in the room, as if part of her was listening for a sound that would never come.

Her children.

She was on remand far from them, and the distance was not just geographic. It was the distance created when the state holds you in a place where you cannot mother, cannot explain, cannot tuck anyone in, cannot make things right with a single phone call.

In the South, separation can be painful. In the Arctic, separation can be a kind of psychic amputation, because the usual bridges are fragile: flights, phones, schedules, permissions, weather. And because in small communities, motherhood is not a private identity. It is woven into who you are to everyone who knows you.

When a mother is held, the whole community feels the absence.

And she feels it most.

DOMESTIC VIOLENCE, COERCION, SURVIVAL STRATEGIES

Her history did not sit neatly under a single label.

If you read the file quickly, you could tell yourself a simple story: she made choices, she broke conditions, she ended up in custody.

But a slower reading, and a slower listening, revealed a more complicated map.

There had been violence in her relationship, but not always in the way the file implied. There were episodes where she was clearly harmed, and episodes where she acted in ways that looked aggressive, but were rooted in a long season of being cornered, emotionally, financially, socially.

Coercion is hard to capture in a police narrative. It doesn't always leave bruises. It leaves restrictions:

- who you can talk to
- where you can go
- how money is controlled
- how your phone is monitored
- how your shame is used as a leash
- how your children become a bargaining chip

When coercion is present, choices take on a different texture. They are still choices, but they happen in a corridor narrowed by fear and dependency.

Sometimes her survival strategies read like contradictions:

- Staying with him, and also trying to leave.
- Calling police, and also refusing to cooperate.
- Speaking, then retracting.
- Agreeing to conditions, then breaching them.

To an outsider, this looks like inconsistency.

To someone who has lived in coercive control, it can be familiar: the mind trying to preserve safety in a world where every option carries danger.

Leaving can be dangerous.

Staying can be dangerous.

Speaking can be dangerous.

Silence can be dangerous.

So people adapt.

They learn to appease. They learn to disappear. They learn to provoke strategically when they want the situation to end quickly. They learn to take the blame because blame is sometimes the cheapest way to stop a conflict from spreading.

And sometimes they learn to use substances, not for pleasure, but for numbness. A way to quiet the nervous system that never fully powers down.

The court sees charges.

The clinician, if careful, sees adaptations.

Not noble adaptations. Not good. Sometimes they are harmful, sometimes unlawful, sometimes destructive.

But still adaptations, developed in a life where control was not evenly distributed.

THE HIDDEN PSYCHIATRIC TOLL OF SEPARATION

The most painful part of remand for her was not the jail.

It was the emptiness created by missing her children.

In custody, people often talk about sleep, food, and boredom. Those are real. But for some mothers, the dominant symptom is something else: a looping grief that doesn't resolve because it cannot be acted on.

Guilt becomes a steady pressure: What are they eating? Are they scared? Do they think I left them? Who is comforting them? What are they hearing about me?

Shame sits beside it: Everyone knows. Everyone will talk. My children will carry my name like a story they didn't choose.

Anxiety fills in the rest: Will I lose them? Will the system decide I'm unfit? Will they be moved? Will they forget me? Will they hate me?

And then, in the quieter hours, depression can arrive, not as sadness, but as a collapse of meaning. Some women don't cry in custody because crying feels unsafe. They go flat. They go silent. They become efficient in the day and hollow at night.

This is the hidden psychiatric toll of separation: the emotional labor of motherhood continues even when the body cannot do mothering.

It becomes a form of suffering that doesn't show up on a risk checklist.

But it shapes everything: motivation, engagement, hope, despair, and sometimes self-harm risk. Not always because the person wants to die, but because the pain of being cut off from their children becomes intolerable.

And in the Arctic, where phone access may be limited and travel may be impossible, separation becomes not only emotional but structural. The absence is reinforced by logistics. The bridge is not just hard to cross. Sometimes it is not there.

THE COURT'S LANGUAGE AND THE MOTHER'S REALITY

The court tends to speak in conditions.

No contact. Curfew. Abstain. Report. Attend. Comply.

For a mother, the reality speaks in needs.

Safety for the children.

Housing that is stable.

Support that is not humiliating.

A plan that doesn't collapse at the first argument.

A way to sleep.

A way to regulate emotions without substances.

A way to be believed without being punished for speaking.

In many cases, a woman in her position is assessed through a lens built for men: the system assumes autonomy, assumes mobility, assumes that just leaving is an option. It often fails to account for the ways dependency, childcare, and coercion shape the real feasibility of compliance.

A condition can be legally reasonable and clinically impossible.

And when it becomes impossible, the predictable result appears in the file as noncompliance, even when the deeper truth is:

She is trying to survive with no stable platform to stand on.

RISK MANAGEMENT VERSUS RECOVERY

When women are held on remand, risk management is often framed narrowly: will she breach again, will she use substances, will she return to the relationship, will there be another incident?

Those are legitimate questions.

But recovery requires a broader frame:

- What does safety look like for her and for the children?
- What does she need to break coercive patterns?
- What supports exist that won't disappear when the circuit plane leaves?
- What is the plan for the first week after release: sleep, food, childcare, check-ins, safe contact points?
- Who will help her navigate the social consequences in a small community where privacy is thin?

If those questions are not answered, the system can release her with conditions that look strict and then act surprised when she returns, breached, exhausted, ashamed, more tangled than before.

That cycle is particularly cruel for mothers because every cycle risks widening the distance between her and her children.

Not just emotionally.

Legally.

Practically.

Permanently.

WHAT I TRIED TO DO IN THE ROOM

In the interview room, I did not try to rescue her. That is not my role, and it is a dangerous fantasy in forensic work.

What I tried to do was slower and more basic:

- Clarify what I was asked to assess
- Name confidentiality limits plainly
- Allow her to speak without forcing a clean narrative
- Ask about coercion without implying blame
- Ask about the children without turning the interview into a sentimental plea
- Assess symptoms honestly: anxiety, trauma responses, depressive features, sleep disruption, substance use patterns
- Identify what would actually reduce risk, real supports, not paper rules

Sometimes, the most therapeutic act available in a forensic setting is accuracy: describing the person's situation in a way that prevents the system from mislabeling survival as defiance.

Accuracy does not undo harm.

But it can reduce future harm, especially the harm created by unrealistic plans.

THE SENTENCE THAT STAYED WITH ME

Near the end of the interview, she said something quietly, without drama, that stayed with me longer than most dramatic statements ever do:

"I don't know how to be a mom from here."

That sentence was not only sadness. It was disorientation.

Because motherhood is not a feeling. It is a routine. A thousand small acts. In custody, those acts are taken away, and the identity becomes painful because it cannot be performed.

When I left that room, I carried the familiar tension of circuit work:

The court wants clarity.

The file wants resolution.

The system wants conditions.

But the person wants something simpler and harder:

A way back to her children that does not guarantee another collapse.

In the Arctic, where distance amplifies everything, that is not just a personal hope.

It is a structural challenge.

And it is one of the most honest measures of justice we rarely name: whether the system can hold accountability and safety without turning separation into a slow, irreversible punishment for families who were already living on the edge.

CHAPTER 25

The Elder With Cognitive Decline in the Justice System

He should not have looked like "a problem."

He was an Elder, quiet, weathered, dignified in the way some people are dignified even when they are frightened. He held himself with a kind of restraint that made others assume he was in control.

But control is not the same as capacity.

By the time he entered the justice system, the problem was not only the alleged offence. The problem was that the system did not know how to recognize cognitive decline when it arrived wearing the face of age, pride, and silence.

MISINTERPRETATION OF CONFUSION AS DEFIANCE

The file described him in familiar institutional language:

- Uncooperative.
- Doesn't follow instructions.
- Refuses to answer.
- Argumentative.
- Noncompliant.

Those words are efficient. They help a system move.

They can also be wrong.

When I met him, I noticed the pauses first. Not dramatic pauses, small delays between question and answer, as if the question needed to travel a longer distance inside his mind before it could be unpacked.

His answers sometimes fit. Sometimes they did not. He could speak clearly about a childhood memory, then lose the thread of what had happened last week. He would agree to something and then look startled when the next question assumed he remembered what he had agreed to. He seemed embarrassed when he could not find words, and in that embarrassment I saw something important: he still had enough insight to feel shame.

Shame is one of the ways cognitive decline hides itself in public.

In court and custody settings, confusion often gets interpreted as disrespect.

Not looking at the judge becomes "attitude."

Not answering quickly becomes "evasive."

Not following directions becomes "deliberate."

Repeating questions becomes "manipulative."

Changing the story becomes "lying."

But cognitive decline can do all of those things without intent.

When you are confused and frightened, you may argue, not because you are defiant, but because arguing is the last tool you have to keep your dignity intact. When you cannot remember, you may insist, because insisting is how you protect yourself from looking weak. When you feel ashamed, you may withdraw, because silence is safer than exposure.

In a small community, an Elder may feel this even more sharply: status and respect matter, and cognitive decline can feel like losing your place in the social world.

So the Elder becomes "difficult."

And the system responds with control.

Which makes the confusion worse.

CAPACITY: THE QUIET QUESTION BEHIND THE LOUD PROCESS

Once cognitive decline enters the room, "capacity" becomes the quiet question behind everything else.

Capacity is not a single trait. It is task-specific, time-specific, and vulnerable to stress. An Elder might be capable of some decisions and not others. Capable on a calm day and not capable after a sleepless night in remand. Capable in their own language at home and not capable under cross-examination through an interpreter in a formal room.

The justice system often asks for crisp answers:

Fit or unfit.

Competent or not.

Responsible or not.

Release or detain.

Cognitive decline rarely offers crispness.

So the clinical work becomes careful, practical, and plain-language:

- Can he understand the basic roles in court?

- Can he follow the thread of a conversation long enough to give meaningful instructions to counsel?
- Can he appreciate consequences in a way that is real, not rote?
- Can he comply with conditions, or will "compliance" become a predictable failure because memory and executive function are impaired?
- Is he vulnerable to suggestion, agreeing just to end the questioning?
- Does he understand his rights?
- Does he understand what he is being asked to do when he signs a document or accepts a plan?

The hardest part is that capacity can be artificially lowered by the environment.

Remand worsens sleep.

Sleep worsens confusion.

Confusion increases agitation.

Agitation increases restriction.

Restriction increases disorientation.

A spiral begins, and the system may mistake the spiral for personality.

VULNERABILITY: WHEN THE SYSTEM BECOMES A RISK FACTOR

Elders with cognitive impairment are vulnerable in custody in ways that are easy to overlook.

They may be bullied or exploited.

They may give away commissary items because they cannot navigate the social rules of jail.

They may miss meals because they are disoriented about routine.

They may become dehydrated.

They may misinterpret staff instructions and then be disciplined for failing.

They may become frightened and aggressive, not out of malice, but out of panic.

They may become depressed quickly, not simply because jail is unpleasant, but because dislocation can be devastating for someone whose orientation depends on familiar cues and familiar people.

And in remote settings, where transfers to specialized care can be delayed by weather or bed shortages, an Elder can remain in a place that is functionally unsafe for them, even if everyone is trying their best.

Sometimes the most honest clinical statement is this:

Custody itself is worsening the condition we are being asked to evaluate.

ALTERNATIVES TO CUSTODY: THE PART OF THE REPORT THAT MATTERS MOST

When an Elder with cognitive decline enters the justice system, the question is not only: What happened?

It is: What is the least harmful way to respond, while still protecting safety and honoring accountability?

Accountability still matters. Harm still matters. Victims still matter. Community trust matters.

But the response must fit the person's capacity and vulnerability, or the system will create new harm that exceeds the harm it is trying to address.

In practice, alternatives to custody often depend on creativity and local coordination:

- Supervised community placement with family or trusted supports, if safe and stable
- Health-center follow-up with clear written instructions and supported attendance
- Simplified conditions (few, concrete, repeatable), recognizing memory limits
- Regular check-ins through a consistent contact person
- Home-based supports where available, rather than expecting travel and appointments that will be missed
- Guardianship or substitute decision-making pathways when appropriate and legally supported
- Medical assessment and treatment planning, including dementia workup when feasible
- Culturally grounded supports that help maintain dignity and reduce disorientation

The essential principle is realism. Conditions must be executable by a person with impaired memory and executive function. Otherwise, the system will manufacture breaches and call them choices.

If the court is going to impose rules, those rules must be rules the person can actually remember.

THE MORAL DISCOMFORT OF LABELING

There is a particular moral discomfort in writing about Elders.

The justice system is designed around adult autonomy: people who can plan, understand, decide, and comply. Cognitive decline exposes how fragile that assumption is.

It also exposes how quickly systems can slide into moral labeling:

"Stubborn."

"Difficult."

"Noncompliant."

"Manipulative."

Sometimes, those words are used because staff are exhausted and trying to keep order.

But in cases of cognitive decline, those labels can become a second injury, an institutional misrecognition that strips dignity.

So I learned to write differently.

To describe observable impairments rather than moral traits.

To distinguish refusal from inability.

To be explicit about how stress, sleep loss, withdrawal, and confinement can worsen cognition.

To recommend alternatives that reduce risk and reduce harm.

And to name, plainly, the central ethical truth:

When the system treats cognitive decline like defiance, it becomes part of the problem.

THE QUIET TRAGEDY AND THE QUIET RESPONSIBILITY

The Elder I am describing here is a composite, but the pattern is real enough that it feels familiar across files and communities.

An older person enters the system late in life, not because they suddenly "became criminal," but because their cognition is slipping, their supports are thinning, and the world is becoming harder to navigate. Confusion shows up as conflict. Conflict shows up as police contact. Police contact shows up as charges. Charges show up as remand.

And remand accelerates the decline.

In the Arctic, where distance slows access to specialized geriatric and neurocognitive care, the system's responsibility becomes sharper. It must not turn scarcity into punishment.

Because if we cannot offer perfect solutions, we can still offer something essential:

A response that recognizes vulnerability as vulnerability, and refuses to confuse confusion with defiance, especially when the person in front of us is an Elder whose dignity should not be collateral damage in the machinery of the process.

PART VII

SYSTEMS, ETHICS, AND THE EDGES OF POWER

CHAPTER 26

When the System Asks for Certainty

The courtroom likes clean lines.

Guilty or not guilty.

Fit or unfit.

High risk or low risk.

Detain or release.

Reliable or not reliable.

It is not that the justice system is intellectually naïve. Judges and lawyers understand complexity better than the public often assumes. But the system is built to make decisions, and decisions require endpoints. The court cannot live forever in "maybe." At some point, it must choose an outcome, and outcomes are often binary.

Forensic psychiatry, meanwhile, lives in gradients.

People are complex. Memories are imperfect. Trauma distorts narrative. Intoxication blurs chronology. Psychosis can come and go. Cognitive functioning can vary day to day. Culture and language shape expression. Risk rises and falls with context. Even diagnosis, often treated as a stable label, is sometimes provisional, evolving, contingent.

So, when the system asks for certainty, it is not always asking for truth.

It is asking for decidability.

And that can create pressure, subtle or overt, for the psychiatrist to sound more certain than the data allows.

PRESSURES IN COURT: YES/NO ANSWERS FOR COMPLEX HUMANS

The pressure begins with the structure of questions. Cross-examination is built to narrow. It takes a person's complexity and pushes it through a funnel until what comes out fits a legal category. That is not necessarily malicious; it is the nature of advocacy. But it can be dangerous if the clinician forgets that the funnel is not the whole story.

"Doctor, is he psychotic, yes or no?"

"Doctor, was he able to understand his actions, yes or no?"

"Doctor, is she at risk of violence, yes or no?"

"Doctor, can he comply with conditions, yes or no?"

"Doctor, can we trust what she said, yes or no?"

These questions contain an implicit demand: choose a side.

In the Arctic, that demand can feel even sharper because time is tight. Circuit days are compressed. Dockets are crowded. People have flown in to be present. There is urgency in the room, sometimes the visible urgency of weather and scheduling, sometimes the hidden urgency of remand harm. Everyone wants the case to move.

And in that urgency, nuance can feel like obstruction.

There is also a quieter pressure. In small systems, people know each other. The court staff, lawyers, and local professionals have ongoing relationships. A visiting expert can feel, without anyone saying it, that a "clean" answer will be easier for everyone.

But forensic integrity is not about ease.

It is about accuracy.

Accuracy is sometimes uncomfortable.

THE TEMPTATION: FALSE CERTAINTY AS PERFORMANCE

False certainty is seductive because it looks like competence. A confident opinion sounds professional. A firm conclusion sounds helpful. A crisp risk label sounds decisive. In a courtroom, decisiveness can be rewarded. It feels like clarity, and clarity feels like control.

But false certainty is not clarity.

It is performance.

And the cost of performance can be high, especially in the Arctic, where the consequences of decisions echo through small communities and where resources are thin. A confident but wrong conclusion can lead to:

- Unnecessary detention
- Unsafe release plans
- Conditions that will predictably fail
- Missed treatment opportunities
- Unjust legal outcomes
- Increased future harm

In forensic work, certainty should not be used to soothe the system's anxiety. The system can tolerate uncertainty if you communicate it well. What it cannot tolerate is vagueness.

So the challenge is not to avoid uncertainty. The challenge is to frame it in a way that remains usable.

COMMUNICATING UNCERTAINTY WITHOUT LOSING CLARITY

Over time, I learned a discipline that feels almost paradoxical:

Be precise about what you know, and equally precise about what you do not.

Uncertainty becomes dangerous when it is sloppy. It becomes ethical when it is structured.

1) *Separate Facts, Inferences, and Opinions*

In court, I learned to make distinctions explicit:

- **Facts:** what was observed, what was reported, what collateral sources documented
- **Inferences:** what those facts suggest, with stated assumptions
- **Opinions:** the clinical conclusion, grounded in the above

This prevents the system from treating interpretation as evidence.

2) *Use Probability Language That Has Meaning*

Instead of "I am not sure," I learned to say:

- "The evidence supports X more strongly than Y."
- "It is more likely than not that…"

- "There is insufficient evidence to conclude…"
- "This conclusion depends on…"
- "If collateral confirms A, then B becomes more likely."

Judges can work with conditional reasoning. They do it all the time. What they need is clarity about conditions.

3) *Anchor Uncertainty in Why It Exists*

Uncertainty is not a personal flaw. It often arises from identifiable limitations:

- Language barriers and interpretation constraints
- Intoxication obscuring recall
- Lack of collateral
- Time-limited assessment due to circuit schedule
- Fluctuating symptoms
- Inconsistent documentation
- Cultural differences in expression
- Environmental effects of remand on mental state

When you name the reason for uncertainty, it becomes credible rather than evasive.

4) *Offer Ranges and Scenarios, Not Hedges*

Courtrooms hate hedges like "maybe" and "it depends" unless you make "depends" concrete.

So instead of "It depends."

You say: "Risk is higher if the person returns to the same household with ongoing alcohol use and conflict, and lower if there is stable housing, structured follow-up, and managed substance use."

That is not vagueness. That is a usable risk formulation.

5) *Translate Clinical Nuance Into Legal Relevance*

The system is not asking for a textbook. It is asking:

- What does this mean for fitness today?
- What does this mean for responsibility at the time?
- What does this mean for risk on release?
- What does this mean for appropriate disposition?

So, uncertainty must be linked to decision points:

- "I cannot conclude X, but I can conclude Y."
- "I cannot speak to intent with certainty, but I can speak to capacity and symptom burden."
- "I cannot predict violence in a binary way, but I can identify predictable triggers and protective factors."

Clarity is not certainty. Clarity is structure.

THE ARCTIC'S SPECIAL TENSION: LIMITED OPTIONS AMPLIFY THE NEED FOR HONESTY

In remote settings, the system's desire for certainty can intensify because there are fewer options. If there were endless programs, abundant beds, and rapid follow-up, uncertainty would feel less frightening. The system could experiment: try one plan, adjust quickly.

But in the Arctic, plans are harder to adjust. Transfers take time. Supports are thin. One decision can set a course that is difficult to change.

That makes honesty even more important.

When the options are limited, the temptation is to force the complexity into a clean conclusion so the system can move forward. But forcing complexity into a simple answer can produce a plan that fails, and failure in the North is costly.

So the ethical response is not to offer certainty. It is to offer a clear map of uncertainty and to help the court choose the least harmful path within that map.

THE QUIET COURAGE OF SAYING "I DON'T KNOW"

There is a kind of quiet courage required to say, in a courtroom, "I don't know," and to say it in a way that still helps. Not because ignorance is virtuous, but because honesty is.

A visiting forensic psychiatrist can be especially tempted to overstate conclusions. You are a guest expert; the system has flown you in; your presence implies that you will resolve ambiguity. It can feel embarrassing to admit limits.

But limits are part of the truth.

And the court does not need a flawless expert. It needs a reliable one.

So I learned to treat uncertainty as part of my professional integrity, not a threat to it. To remember that the goal is not to sound certain. The goal is to be accurate and to communicate accuracy in a form the court can use.

Because complex humans do not become simple just because a courtroom prefers clean answers.

And in the Arctic, where decisions echo loudly in small communities, the cost of pretending otherwise is too high.

CHAPTER 27

Cultural Safety in Forensic Practice

In the North, culture is not a "factor." Culture is the air people breathe.

And when you arrive as a visiting forensic psychiatrist, carrying the court's questions, the institution's expectations, and your own training, you are also carrying something else: a framework that can easily become an instrument of harm if you are not careful.

Cultural safety in forensic practice is not a checklist. It is not a paragraph you add to a report. It is not a polite nod to tradition.

It is the daily discipline of asking: Am I practicing in a way that reduces harm, respects lived realities, and does not reproduce the power dynamics that have injured communities for generations?

That discipline matters doubly in forensic contexts, because your words do not stay in the room. They become part of the legal record. They travel through systems. They can be used to justify decisions that affect liberty, family, and community safety.

So cultural safety is not optional.

It is part of competence.

AVOIDING PATHOLOGIZING CULTURE

One of the most common errors visiting clinicians make is treating cultural difference as clinical abnormality.

Not intentionally. Often unconsciously.

A person speaks less, and the clinician interprets it as guardedness, poor insight, or suspiciousness, when it may be respectful restraint.

A person avoids eye contact, and the clinician interprets it as evasiveness, when it may be a sign of respect.

A person describes spiritual experiences, and the clinician interprets them as hallucinations, when they may be culturally normative, meaningful, and not associated with impairment.

A person answers indirectly, and the clinician interprets it as manipulation, when it may be a culturally shaped communication style.

A person's distress is expressed somatically through pain, fatigue, or heaviness, and the clinician interprets it as "lack of psychological insight," rather than a legitimate idiom of distress.

In forensic settings, these misinterpretations are dangerous because they can inflate psychopathology and inflate risk. They can lead to diagnostic conclusions that carry stigma and legal consequences.

Cultural safety requires a disciplined pause before labeling:

- Is this behavior actually a symptom, or is it a norm in this context?
- Is this belief actually delusional, or is it culturally shared and non-impairing?
- Is this silence avoidance, or is it a respectful way of holding emotion?
- Is this narrative fragmented because of deceit, or because trauma and shame shape how stories are told?
- Is this "noncompliance," or is it a mismatch between conditions and lived realities?

The safest forensic posture is not to assume you understand.

It is to assume you might be misunderstanding and to check.

AVOIDING ROMANTICIZING SUFFERING

The second common error is the opposite: romanticizing.

The North can seduce visitors into aesthetic narratives: resilience, beauty, tradition, strength, survival. Those are real truths. But when a clinician leans too hard into them, they can become a way of avoiding the harder truths: structural scarcity, violence exposure, colonial harms, service gaps, and the daily stressors that shape mental health and justice involvement.

Romanticizing suffering is a subtle form of disrespect.

It turns hardship into story.

It can make poverty sound poetic.

It can make trauma sound like character-building.

It can make systemic failure sound like "a different way of life."

Cultural safety requires holding both truths at once:

- Honoring cultural strengths and protective practices
- While naming, plainly, the structural harms that increase risk and suffering

In forensic writing, this matters because romanticizing can lead to minimization: "They're resilient, they'll be fine," when the person is actually at high risk of relapse, violence, or self-harm due to unaddressed needs.

The ethical stance is neither pathologizing nor romanticizing.

It is realism with respect.

CULTURAL SAFETY IN THE INTERVIEW ROOM

Cultural safety begins before the first question.

It begins with how you introduce yourself, how you frame your role, how you explain confidentiality limits, how you acknowledge the context of court involvement.

In many Indigenous communities, the justice system is not seen as neutral. There are historical reasons for mistrust and contemporary reasons too. A visiting clinician is easily perceived as part of the state's machinery, even when their intent is compassionate.

So the first task is transparency:

- Why you are there?
- Who asked for the assessment?
- What you will do with the information?
- What will and will not remain confidential?
- How the report may be used?
- What the person's choices are within the process?

Then comes pacing.

In some contexts, rapid-fire questioning feels invasive and unsafe. Time matters. Silence matters. Allowing story to unfold matters. But so does structure, because forensic work cannot become a free-floating conversation. The art is to be structured without being coercive.

And then comes language.

If interpretation is used, cultural safety includes respecting the interpreter's role, ensuring meaning is not smoothed over, and recognizing that some concepts do not translate neatly into English psychiatric categories.

CULTURAL SAFETY IN FORMULATION

Formulation is where cultural safety becomes real.

A diagnosis can be technically "correct" and still culturally unsafe if it ignores context, ignores idioms of distress, and ignores the power dynamics that shape behavior.

A culturally safe formulation asks:

- What happened to this person?
- What stressors are ongoing?
- What cultural and community strengths exist?
- What supports are realistically available here?
- How do historical and structural factors shape present risk and coping?
- How might my own assumptions be shaping what I see as "symptoms"?

It also requires attention to what not to do:

- Do not equate culture with risk
- Do not imply that "Indigenousness" explains violence or addiction
- Do not treat historical trauma as a universal excuse or a universal diagnosis
- Do not assume that Western treatment is the only legitimate pathway to change

Cultural safety does not mean avoiding diagnosis. It means ensuring the diagnosis is not a blunt instrument.

CONSULTATION WITH COMMUNITY KNOWLEDGE HOLDERS (WHERE APPROPRIATE)

In forensic practice, consultation must be handled carefully.

There are ethical and legal constraints: confidentiality, boundaries, role clarity, and the risk of putting community members in difficult positions. Not every case is appropriate for consultation with community knowledge holders, and it should never be done casually.

But where appropriate, and where consent, confidentiality safeguards, and role clarity can be maintained, consultation can improve accuracy and reduce harm.

Community knowledge holders may include Elders, cultural advisors, local wellness workers, or others recognized for cultural expertise. Their contribution is not to decide legal outcomes or diagnose mental illness. Their contribution is to help a visiting clinician understand:

- Culturally normative beliefs and practices
- Local idioms of distress and healing
- Historical context relevant to trust and engagement
- Culturally grounded supports that could be protective
- The realities of service access and what "treatment" actually looks like locally

In practical terms, culturally safe consultation requires:

- Explicit consent from the person being assessed (where the consultation relates to their case)

- Clear boundaries about what will be discussed and what will not
- Respectful compensation or recognition where appropriate (without tokenism)
- Documentation that reflects consultation appropriately without exposing confidential community information
- Awareness of dual relationships in small communities; consultation should not place a knowledge holder in harm's way socially or emotionally

Sometimes, consultation is not possible. Sometimes it would be unsafe. Cultural safety then requires something simpler: humility, careful interpretation, and avoiding assumptions.

THE GOAL: ACCURACY WITHOUT HARM

Cultural safety in forensic psychiatry is not about being "nice."

It is about being accurate without causing unnecessary harm. A culturally unsafe assessment can mislabel, misinterpret, and magnify risk unfairly.

A culturally safe assessment can still conclude that someone is high risk, still acknowledge serious harm, and still recommend restrictions when necessary, but it does so with language and reasoning that respects context and avoids stereotypes.

It says, in effect:

- This person is responsible for their actions
- This community's history matters
- This system's limitations matter

- This culture is not a pathology
- This suffering is not a story to be romanticized
- And this report will aim to reduce harm, not add to it

In the North, that is the ethical minimum.

And for a visiting forensic psychiatrist, it is also the only way to deserve the trust you are asking for, briefly, imperfectly, but with intention, when you enter a place that has every reason to be cautious of outsiders who arrive with authority.

CHAPTER 28

Moral Injury and the Limits of "One Visit"

The plane always leaves.

No matter how heavy the docket was. No matter how many people were still waiting. No matter how many files remained open, how many "follow-ups" were written in the margins, how many voices stayed in my head after I closed the laptop.

The plane always leaves, and the visitor always becomes a departure.

In the South, leaving at the end of the day is ordinary. In the Arctic, leaving is an ethical event. It is a reminder that your presence was temporary, that your authority was borrowed, and that whatever you recommended may or may not survive the gap between what should happen and what can happen.

That gap is where moral injury lives.

LEAVING WHEN NEEDS REMAIN

In medicine, we talk a lot about burnout, fatigue, workload, emotional exhaustion.

Moral injury is different.

Moral injury is what happens when you are asked to participate in a system that cannot reliably do what you know is needed, and you cannot fix it from inside your role. It is the distress of knowing the right thing and being unable to deliver it, not because you do not care, not because you lack skill, but because the infrastructure is thin and the consequences of thinness fall on human beings.

On circuit, the injury was often quiet.

It was not a dramatic crisis. It was the ordinary accumulation of unfinished care:

- The person with emerging psychosis who needed stable follow-up, but would return to a community with intermittent services
- The woman on remand who needed trauma-informed support, but would be released into the same coercive environment
- The young man with ADHD and addiction who needed structure and treatment, but would receive conditions and then be breached
- The Elder with cognitive decline who needed assessment and safer placement, but might remain in custody because alternatives were scarce

You could feel it in the way people asked questions at the end of interviews:

- "So what happens now?"
- "Will you be back?"
- "Are you the only doctor?"
- "Can you help me get out?"
- "Can you tell them I'm not crazy?"
- "Can you tell them I need to see my kids?"

Those questions carry hope, and hope can be dangerous when you cannot meet it.

As a visiting forensic psychiatrist, you have to be honest. You cannot promise continuity you cannot provide. You cannot promise programs that do not exist. You cannot promise timelines the weather can break.

But honesty does not protect you from the feeling of leaving when needs remain.

In fact, honesty can make it worse.

Because you see the person's face when they realize that "help" might be a report, not a relationship.

And in forensic work, a report can be powerful, but it is also impersonal.

It does not sit with someone on the night they cannot sleep.

It does not answer the phone when cravings rise.

It does not de-escalate the argument before it becomes another police call.

It does not pick someone up for an appointment when the taxi money is gone.

It sits in a file.

And the person remains in a life.

THE BURDEN OF RECOMMENDATIONS THAT CANNOT BE IMPLEMENTED LOCALLY

Forensic reports often end with recommendations. That is part of their shape: assessment, formulation, risk, recommendations.

In the South, recommending is easier. You can recommend a program and know it exists. You can recommend outpatient follow-up and assume the referral will land somewhere. You can recommend medication monitoring and know labs can be done. You can recommend psychotherapy and assume there is a therapist within reach.

In the Arctic, recommending can feel like writing letters to a future that may not arrive.

You find yourself adding qualifiers:

- "Where available"
- "If resources allow"
- "Subject to staffing"
- "Contingent on transfer"
- "Consider if feasible"

Those phrases keep the report honest, but they also reveal the truth: the recommendation is not a plan. It is a wish shaped into professional language.

And then there is the other burden: recommendations can create expectations.

A judge may expect follow-up to happen because the report says it should.

A probation plan may include treatment attendance because the report recommended it.

Conditions may be built around services that are intermittent.

When the services fail to materialize, the person can be blamed for not following through.

So the visiting psychiatrist becomes, without intending it, a contributor to the breach cycle.

That is a hard thing to hold.

It forces a deeper discipline: in remote settings, you must recommend only what is realistically possible, or you must recommend with explicit contingency plans that prevent impossibility from becoming blame.

That discipline can feel like compromise.

But it is not a compromise of ethics. It is ethical realism.

"ONE VISIT" AS A STRUCTURAL LIMITATION

The phrase "one visit" sounds simple. It implies a single clinical encounter.

In the Arctic, "one visit" is not just an appointment. It is a structural limitation imposed by geography, staffing, and the way services are organized.

One visit means:

- You meet someone at a crisis point
- You gather what you can quickly
- You offer what you can in a report
- And then you leave before the story moves forward

This changes your relationship to uncertainty. It changes your relationship to the people you assess. It changes your relationship to your own conscience.

Because the work is incomplete by design.

You do not get to see what happens after your recommendation.

You do not get to adjust when the plan fails.

You do not get to repair ruptures in trust.

You do not get to hold continuity.

You leave behind words.

And in a system starved of continuity, words can feel both powerful and painfully insufficient.

THE QUIET WAYS MORAL INJURY SHOWS UP

Moral injury does not always arrive as tears or breakdown.

Often it arrives as small, repeatable sensations:

- A heaviness in the chest when you close the file
- A restless night after a day of custody interviews
- An irritation you do not recognize as grief
- A sense of guilt that feels irrational but is not
- A moment of dread when you hear that the same person is back on the docket again
- A reluctance to recommend because you already know the recommendation will not hold
- A cynicism that threatens to replace compassion

The danger is that moral injury can harden a clinician.

It can make you stop caring, not because you are cruel, but because caring without capacity to help can feel unbearable.

The Arctic taught me that hardening is not professionalism.

It is injury.

WHAT HELPED: A DIFFERENT KIND OF INTEGRITY

I learned that the antidote to moral injury is not optimism.

It is integrity.

Integrity, in this context, means:

- Writing recommendations that are realistic and specific
- Naming system limitations plainly, so the burden does not fall invisibly on the person
- Building contingency into plans ("if X is not available, then Y")
- Collaborating closely with local staff who know what can actually happen
- Respecting cultural and community strengths rather than imposing southern models
- Accepting that you cannot solve structural scarcity with personal effort
- Finding ways to stay human without pretending you can be everything

It also means allowing yourself to feel the discomfort without rushing to numb it.

Because the discomfort is evidence that your ethics are still alive.

THE DEPARTURE

On the morning of departure, the rituals were simple: a bag packed, a check-out, a taxi, the airport, the familiar cold.

But inside, the departure was never simple.

Leaving meant carrying names and faces and stories that would continue without you.

Leaving meant trusting local colleagues to do the work you could not stay to do.

Leaving meant knowing that some people would improve and some would deteriorate, and you might never know which.

Leaving meant accepting that the limits of "one visit" are not your personal failure, but they still produce a personal ache.

That ache is moral injury's quiet signature.

It is the cost of trying to practice humane forensic psychiatry in a place where the needs are real and the resources are finite.

And it is also, strangely, what keeps you returning.

Because even when one visit is not enough, it is sometimes still better than no visit at all, not as a justification for scarcity, not as a comfort for the system, but as a small, imperfect act of presence in a geography that makes presence hard.

The plane always leaves.

But the stories remain.

CHAPTER 29

Evacuation Decisions

In the Arctic, there are moments when the most important clinical decision is not a diagnosis or a medication. It is a flight.

Evacuation, being flown south for assessment or treatment, sounds clinical, even procedural. The word carries a tone of efficiency: a transport decision, a transfer, a referral. In practice, evacuation is one of the most consequential interventions a northern system can make, because it is never only medical.

It is geographic.

It is cultural.

It is relational.

It is identity-altering.

And for the person being moved, it can feel like being uprooted from the last pieces of familiarity at the moment they are least able to tolerate dislocation.

WHEN SOMEONE MUST BE FLOWN SOUTH

Sometimes, evacuation is clearly indicated.

A person is acutely psychotic and unsafe, and local resources cannot provide the level of care required.

A person is severely suicidal, and the local environment cannot safely contain the risk without causing further harm.

A person is delirious, medically unstable, or in complicated withdrawal, and local medical capacity is limited.

A person's cognitive state is collapsing, and the workup needed cannot be done locally.

A person's violence risk is escalating beyond what custody or local health services can manage safely.

In these moments, the choice is not between "staying" and "going" as equal options. The choice is between a flawed local containment and a higher level of care that exists only elsewhere.

But even when evacuation is clinically necessary, it is never simple.

Because the decision carries two kinds of risk:

- The risk of staying without adequate care
- The risk of leaving and causing rupture

The art is not pretending one risk disappears. The art is deciding which risk is more ethically tolerable, given what is happening in front of you.

THE THRESHOLD: NOT ONLY ILLNESS, BUT CAPACITY TO CARE

In southern systems, the threshold for transfer is often primarily clinical: acuity, safety, diagnostic uncertainty, need for specialized interventions.

In the Arctic, the threshold is also logistical and institutional:

- Do we have enough staff to provide safe observation?
- Is there a safe space that is not segregation?

- Can we administer and monitor necessary medications?
- Can we manage severe withdrawal?
- Can we provide culturally safe care?
- Can we keep this person, and others, safe without escalating harm?

Sometimes the person's clinical condition is serious but might be manageable with adequate supports. The evacuation becomes necessary because those supports are not reliably available.

In those moments, the evacuation decision becomes a reflection of system capacity as much as individual pathology.

That is one of its moral burdens.

The cost of distance.

Evacuation is not just travel. It is a rupture.

THERAPEUTIC RUPTURE

If the person has any local relationships—a nurse they trust, a community worker who knows their story, an Elder who has spoken to them, even a corrections officer whose consistency has calmed them—evacuation breaks that thread.

In the receiving hospital, the person becomes a stranger again. Their story is retold in fragments. Their cultural context may be misunderstood. Their coping strategies may be misread. Their language may not be shared. Their supports are far.

Even the most skilled southern team cannot replicate local familiarity. And in mental health care, familiarity can be stabilizing.

A person who was just beginning to trust may shut down.

A person who was barely holding together may unravel in the unfamiliarity.

Evacuation can save a life and still injure trust.

IDENTITY

For many people, especially Indigenous people, identity is not an individual abstraction. It is rooted in land, kinship, language, and community roles.

To be flown south in a state of crisis can feel like being removed not only from a place, but from oneself.

Some people describe it like exile.

Even when the intention is care, the experience can echo historical patterns of removal, children taken, people sent away, decisions made by institutions far from home. That echo matters. It can intensify fear and resistance. It can activate trauma in ways that complicate treatment.

The person may interpret transfer not as help, but as punishment.

Not because they are irrational, but because history has taught communities to be cautious of distant systems that claim benevolence while exerting control.

FAMILY DISRUPTION

Evacuation disrupts families in the bluntest way: distance.

Families may not be able to travel. The cost is too high. The flights are too rare. The logistics are too complex. The family may not have childcare for other children. They may not have leave from work. They may not feel safe travelling. They may not feel welcome in southern settings.

So the person is hospitalized without family presence.

Phone contact may be limited or inconsistent.

Information flow becomes strained.

For a parent, the disruption can be devastating, especially if they fear child welfare involvement, or if they are already struggling with shame and anxiety.

For an Elder, the dislocation can worsen confusion and depression.

For anyone, the loneliness can amplify symptoms.

In the South, we sometimes underestimate how much family presence stabilizes people. In the Arctic, family absence is not a side effect. It is part of the intervention.

And it carries psychiatric consequences.

EVACUATION FROM CUSTODY: DOUBLE DISLOCATION

Evacuation decisions become even more complex when the person is in custody.

Now the dislocation is doubled:

- From community to the South
- And from liberty to custody constraints

There may be escorts, restraints, and security protocols. The person's dignity is tested at every step. The transfer can feel like punishment even when it is medical. The hospital environment may still be locked, still guarded, still controlled.

A person who is already paranoid may interpret the transfer as confirmation of persecution.

A person with trauma may experience it as a reenactment of capture and removal.

A person with cognitive decline may become profoundly disoriented.

The receiving team may inherit not only a patient, but a narrative: "dangerous," "uncooperative," "forensic."

That narrative can shape care, sometimes unfairly.

So the visiting forensic psychiatrist must think not only about the necessity of evacuation, but about how to reduce its harms:

- How is the transfer explained to the person in plain language?
- Is interpretation available?
- Can family be contacted early?
- Can local trusted staff provide a warm handover narrative that humanizes the person?
- Can culturally grounded supports be involved where feasible?
- Can the receiving team be briefed on context so symptoms are not misread?

These small steps cannot erase distance, but they can soften rupture.

THE ETHICAL TENSION: SAVING SOMEONE AND BREAKING SOMETHING

Evacuation is often a decision where you save someone by breaking something.

You may save someone's life by breaking their sense of belonging.

You may stabilize psychosis by breaking a fragile thread of local trust.

You may prevent suicide by breaking family proximity.

You may protect the community by breaking the person's connection to home.

That is not a reason to avoid evacuation when it is needed.

It is a reason to treat evacuation as an ethically heavy intervention, one that requires the same thoughtful consent, explanation, and harm-reduction mindset that we apply to restraint or forced medication.

It should never be framed as "just a flight."

RETURNING: THE NEGLECTED SECOND HALF OF THE STORY

The evacuation story does not end in the southern hospital.

The second half is return.

Return is often where the system fails quietly: discharge plans that assume southern infrastructure, medication regimens that cannot be monitored locally, follow-up appointments that do not exist, referrals that do not land, families who are not prepared, housing that is unstable.

A person can be stabilized in the South and then destabilized on return, not because treatment did not work, but because continuity breaks again.

So an ethically sound evacuation decision includes planning for return:

- Realistic medication choices
- Clear communication with local health centers
- A plan for follow-up that matches local capacity
- Crisis contingencies

- Culturally safe supports where available
- Acknowledgement that the person will need reorientation, not just discharge

In the Arctic, evacuation is often the only viable option for acute care. But if return is not planned, evacuation becomes a revolving door: flown out in crisis, stabilized briefly, flown back into scarcity, and then flown out again when the cycle repeats.

WHAT THE ARCTIC TAUGHT ME

Evacuation decisions taught me that distance is not neutral.

Distance is a clinical variable.

Distance shapes outcomes.

Distance shapes trust.

Distance shapes identity.

And every time the system decides to fly someone south, it is not only transporting a patient.

It is transporting a person away from the networks that make them who they are, at the very moment they are least able to bear disconnection.

That is why evacuation decisions require more than clinical acuity.

They require humility.

They require cultural safety.

They require a harm-reduction approach to dislocation.

And they require remembering what the plane ride always risks erasing:

People do not heal in abstraction.

They heal in places, with people, in relationships.

When we must remove them from those things, we should do it with the seriousness it deserves, because in the Arctic, a flight is never just a flight.

PART VIII

BUILDING BETTER JUSTICE AND BETTER CARE

CHAPTER 30

What Actually Works in the Arctic

If you spend enough time on circuit, you stop asking what should work and start asking what actually holds when the weather turns, the flight cancels, the staffing is thin, and the person is released back into a life with no spare margin.

The Arctic is not a place where theory survives unchanged.

It makes every plan prove itself.

Over time, patterns emerge: quiet successes that do not look dramatic but reduce harm in ways the system can feel: fewer crises, fewer breaches, fewer returns to remand, fewer evacuations that could have been prevented, more stability that lasts longer than a week.

What works in the Arctic tends to share two traits:

1. It is built for interruption, because interruption is normal.
2. It is built around continuity, because continuity is rare and therefore powerful.

STABILIZATION PATHWAYS THAT DO NOT DEPEND ON PERFECT CONDITIONS

The most effective systems I saw did not wait for people to become "ready" or "stable enough" before offering help. They had stabilization pathways: clear, repeatable steps that could be activated quickly when someone was escalating.

Not grand programs. Practical pathways.

- A known place to go when the nervous system is boiling over.
- A known person to call who will answer and understands the local realities.
- A basic protocol for sleep restoration, withdrawal support, and medication continuity.
- A way to reduce chaos for 48 to 72 hours so the person can think again.

In remote settings, the first goal is often not insight.

It is regulation.

Sleep, food, warmth, predictable contact, reduced conflict exposure, and a plan that does not change every day. Those basic things can prevent a spiral from turning into custody or evacuation.

CRISIS ALTERNATIVES THAT FEEL REAL, NOT RHETORICAL

Crisis alternative can sound like policy language. In the Arctic, it has to be concrete.

Because if the only crisis response is police → remand → deterioration, then the system is not responding to crisis. It is recycling it.

What worked best were alternatives that matched local capacity:

- A short-stay, low-barrier stabilization space where available, even a small one with limited hours, that could prevent unnecessary custody.

- A mobile or on-call crisis team model, scaled to reality, sometimes one or two skilled people with clear protocols.
- Agreements between health, justice, and community services about what happens at 2 a.m. when someone is suicidal, psychotic, or withdrawing.

The key was not perfection. It was predictability.

People cope better when they know what will happen next.

LAND-BASED AND CULTURALLY GROUNDED SUPPORTS WHEN THEY ARE TRULY AVAILABLE

Where land-based supports exist, and where they are led and defined by community, not imported as a romantic idea, they can be profoundly stabilizing.

Not because land is magic.

Because land can provide what many people lack: belonging, identity, regulated rhythm, and a way to feel grounded that is not only cognitive or verbal.

For some, land-based supports function as:

- A non-shaming pathway back to routine
- A place where mentorship and accountability can happen naturally
- A context where trauma does not have to be the first language of healing
- A practical alternative to boredom and relapse triggers

The caution is important. Cultural safety means not turning culture into a prescription or a performance. Land-based supports work best when they are offered as real supports: resourced, consistent, and community-held, not as decorative add-ons to an otherwise unchanged system.

CONTINUITY AS THE INTERVENTION

Continuity is the single most effective "treatment" the Arctic can offer, and the hardest to protect.

People do not stabilize because someone had a brilliant idea once. They stabilize because someone stayed connected long enough for change to become possible.

Continuity can look simple:

- One consistent clinician or case-contact
- One consistent court worker or probation officer who knows the person's patterns
- One consistent plan that is repeated and adjusted, not replaced
- One reliable medication list that survives transfers and release
- One follow-up appointment that actually happens, then another

In the North, the system often treats continuity as a luxury.

It is not.

It is the infrastructure of safety.

TELE-FORENSICS AND SHARED CARE THAT RESPECTS LOCAL INTELLIGENCE

Telehealth in the Arctic is not a novelty. It is a necessity. But it works best when it is not used as a cheap substitute for presence.

What actually works is tele-forensics paired with local anchoring:

- The remote specialist provides assessment, formulation, and support.
- Local nurses, wellness workers, court workers, and community teams hold the day-to-day continuity.
- The plan is co-owned, not handed down.

Shared care works when the specialist respects local intelligence, because local staff know what will fail before it fails. They know whose home is safe, what conditions are impossible, what compliance means in that community, and what supports people actually trust.

The best tele-forensic work I have seen is not remote expertise replacing local care.

It is remote expertise strengthening local care.

PRACTICAL FIXES THAT REDUCE BREACHES AND REDUCE REMAND CHURN

The Arctic does not need more clever conditions. It needs fewer impossible ones.

What worked, again and again, were practical fixes that made breach cycles less predictable:

- Simplified conditions: fewer rules, clearer rules, conditions that can be remembered and realistically followed.
- Problem-solving conditions: not just abstain, but what happens when relapse occurs, who is called, what the response is, and how we reduce harm without instantly returning to custody.

- Housing-first realism: recognizing that without a stable place to sleep, most conditions are fantasy.
- Early follow-up windows: prioritizing the first 72 hours after release, including sleep, food, a check-in, and a plan for triggers.
- Interpretation built-in: not as an afterthought, but as part of safety planning and court understanding.

When the system stopped confusing impossibility with defiance, outcomes improved. Not because people became saintly, but because plans began to match the physics of northern life.

PEER SUPPORTS: THE MISSING LAYER THE SYSTEM FORGETS

Professionals matter. Programs matter. Policies matter.

But peer support, where available and properly supported, often changes something professionals cannot: credibility.

A peer can say, “I know what this feels like,” and mean it in a way the system cannot imitate.

Peers can also provide:

- Practical coaching for appointments and routines
- Help navigating shame after court
- Early detection of relapse or escalation
- A non-punitive bridge between crisis and care

In small communities, peer support has to be handled carefully. Privacy, dual relationships, and stigma matter. But when done well, it becomes one of the most scalable forms of continuity, because it is not dependent on specialist scarcity.

A PRINCIPLE THAT REPEATS: BUILD FOR THE ENVIRONMENT, NOT AGAINST IT

The Arctic rewards plans that acknowledge:

- Weather will interrupt
- Staff will turn over
- Phones will fail
- Flights will cancel
- Anonymity is impossible
- Relationships are dense
- Shame travels fast
- Recovery is easier when dignity is protected

So what actually works is often not dramatic innovation. It is design that fits reality:

- Continuity that survives interruption
- Crisis options that are real and reachable
- Culturally grounded supports that are not romanticized
- Tele-forensics that strengthens local care rather than replacing it
- Conditions that can be lived, not only written
- Peer and community supports that keep a person connected after the court day ends

In the end, the Arctic teaches a simple, demanding lesson: If a plan cannot survive Thursday night, it is not a plan.

What works is what holds in the dark, in the cold, after the professionals go home, and sometimes after the plane leaves.

CHAPTER 31

Rethinking Conditions, Remand, and "Risk"

In the justice system, "risk" is often treated like a property of a person.

He is high risk.

She is low risk.

This one cannot be trusted.

That one can be managed in the community.

On circuit, I learned that risk is rarely that simple. Risk is not only inside the person. Risk is also inside the environment, housing, services, family conflict, substance availability, weather, poverty, stigma, and the thinness of follow-up. In the Arctic, those environmental variables are loud. They push and pull on people's behavior the way wind pushes and pulls on a plane.

So if we want fewer breaches, fewer remand spirals, fewer evacuations, and fewer victims harmed, we have to rethink three linked things:

1. Conditions
2. Remand
3. What we mean by "risk"

Because the traditional approach—tighten conditions, increase remand, punish breaches—often produces the opposite of safety in the North. It creates cycles that are predictable, preventable, and expensive in human terms.

DESIGNING REALISTIC BAIL PLANS

A realistic bail plan is not a moral demand. It is engineering. It begins with a simple but neglected question: What can this person actually do, in this place, with the resources they have?

START WITH CAPACITY AND CONTEXT

Before you list conditions, you assess:

- Does the person have stable housing, truly stable, not "a couch that might disappear"?
- Do they have a working phone?
- Can they travel to appointments reliably?
- Do they have childcare responsibilities?
- Do they have cognitive limitations that affect memory and planning?
- Are they in withdrawal or early recovery?
- What triggers violence or relapse in their real life?
- Who are the protective people, and are those relationships functional?
- What services actually exist locally, and how often do they run?

If those realities are not addressed, conditions become aspirational and breaches become predictable.

FEWER CONDITIONS, CLEARER CONDITIONS

In the Arctic, long lists fail. A person with ADHD, trauma, addiction, insomnia, and unstable housing will not manage twelve rules that change their daily behavior. They will forget. They will become overwhelmed. They will default to old patterns. Then the system will call it "noncompliance."

A better approach is:

- Fewer conditions
- Written plainly
- Reviewed with teach-back ("Tell me what this means in your own words.")
- Matched to the person's actual risks

Conditions should be memorable and doable.

AVOID "PAPER SAFETY"

Some conditions look like safety but do not create it:

- Curfews imposed on chaotic, overcrowded homes
- No-contact orders without practical avoidance strategies in a small community
- Abstinence conditions without accessible treatment pathways
- "Attend counselling" when counselling is intermittent or waitlisted
- "Keep the peace" conditions that assume conflict can be prevented by willpower alone

Paper safety creates legal comfort and practical failure. Real safety requires conditions that can be lived.

BUILD THE PLAN AROUND THE FIRST 72 HOURS

The first three days after release are often when risk spikes, relapse occurs, conflict escalates, impulsivity rises, and despair grows. Realistic bail plans prioritize that window:

- Sleep plan
- Food plan
- Safe place to stay
- Check-in plan
- Trigger plan
- Who to call when escalation starts
- What happens if cravings hit at night

A plan that starts on day seven is too late.

HARM REDUCTION AND GRADUATED SUPPORTS INSTEAD OF PUNITIVE CYCLES

The punitive cycle is familiar: Conditions are strict → person breaches → new charges → remand → deterioration → release with stricter conditions → breach again.

It looks like accountability. It often functions like escalation.

Harm reduction is not permissiveness. It is realism about how change happens, especially when addiction, trauma, and scarcity are present.

HARM REDUCTION IN JUSTICE LANGUAGE

A harm-reduction approach asks:

- How do we reduce the chance of serious harm even if relapse or conflict occurs?
- How do we respond to early warning signs without waiting for a breach?
- How do we stabilize rather than punish predictable symptoms of chaos?

For substance use, that might mean:

- Structured check-ins
- Relapse response plans ("If you use, do X immediately; here's who to call")
- Safer-use supports where appropriate
- Medication continuity
- Rapid re-engagement pathways rather than automatic re-incarceration

For violence risk, that might mean:

- Identified de-escalation supports
- Cooling-off plans and safe spaces
- Structured routines that reduce idle time and exposure to triggers
- Realistic no-contact strategies with community-specific logistics
- Immediate support when conflict rises rather than after it explodes

GRADUATED SUPPORTS: CONSEQUENCES AND SCAFFOLDING

Graduated supports do not eliminate accountability. They scale it. They recognize that not every breach is the same. Missing an appointment because the phone died is not the same as stalking a complainant. Drinking once after release is not the same as repeated violent intoxication. Curfew breaches in overcrowded housing are not the same as planned intimidation.

Graduation means:

- Responses proportional to risk
- Early interventions before the spiral becomes a charge
- Consequences paired with increased support, not support removed

The goal is not to excuse. The goal is to stop recycling predictable failure.

REPLACE "BREACH AS CRIME" WITH "BREACH AS SIGNAL"

In many northern cases, breaches are less about criminal intent and more about:

- Executive dysfunction
- Untreated illness
- Addiction relapse
- Unsafe housing
- Unrealistic conditions

Treating every breach as a new crime can turn the justice system into a chronic-stress generator. Chronic stress increases relapse and violence risk. The system then claims it is responding to risk, when it is also producing it.

A smarter approach is to treat many breaches as signals:

- The plan is failing
- Supports are insufficient
- Conditions are unrealistic
- The person is escalating

Then you adjust the plan quickly, rather than waiting for the next charge.

REDEFINING "RISK" IN THE ARCTIC

In the Arctic, "risk" is often a measure of mismatch:

- Mismatch between legal expectations and lived reality
- Mismatch between conditions and housing
- Mismatch between abstinence demands and treatment access
- Mismatch between cognitive capacity and compliance burden
- Mismatch between crisis needs and available services

So a better risk assessment asks:

- What are the predictable risk conditions?
- What can be changed in the environment to reduce risk?
- What supports actually exist locally?
- What is the least restrictive plan that can realistically hold?

- What is the safety plan when the plan starts to fail?

This is not softness. It is precision.

Because the Arctic does not reward pretend control, it rewards plans built for reality.

THE POINT: SAFETY THAT SURVIVES THE REAL WORLD

The goal of rethinking conditions, remand, and risk is not to make the system feel kinder on paper. It is to make the system work.

Work meaning:

- Fewer victims harmed
- Fewer people deteriorating in remand unnecessarily
- Fewer breaches that are predictable and preventable
- Fewer revolving-door evacuations
- More stability that lasts beyond court day

In the North, a bail plan that cannot be lived is a trap.

A response to breach that escalates without support is a factory.

And a concept of "risk" that ignores geography and scarcity is not risk assessment at all. It is storytelling.

If we want better justice and better care, we have to design for the environment we are actually in, not the one our forms assume.

CHAPTER 32

Training and Retention

In the Arctic, the most important clinical intervention is often not a medication, a report, or even a transfer.

It is staying power.

Not the visiting specialist's staying power, because the plane will always leave, but the system's capacity to keep skilled people in place long enough for continuity to become normal, not exceptional.

Training and retention are usually discussed as workforce issues. On circuit, I came to see them as safety issues.

Because every time a nurse leaves, a relationship breaks.

Every time a court worker burns out, a bridge collapses.

Every time a probation officer rotates out, a plan resets to zero.

Every time a visiting psychiatrist arrives without local anchoring, the community is asked to adjust to a new voice, a new style, a new set of assumptions.

In the North, turnover doesn't just reduce service quality.

It multiplies risk.

So if we want better justice and better care, we have to treat training and retention as part of the clinical system, not as an administrative problem happening somewhere else.

SUPPORTING LOCAL STAFF

Local staff are the spine of northern systems: nurses, social workers, wellness workers, court workers, probation officers, victim services staff, corrections officers, interpreters, and community knowledge holders.

They carry responsibilities that would be distributed across multiple teams in the South. They do crisis work, coordination, de-escalation, paperwork, informal counselling, and "relationship repair" inside a system that breaks relationships by design.

Supporting them requires more than telling them they are appreciated.

It requires building structures that reduce moral injury and make the work sustainable.

1) *Predictable Clinical Backup*

One of the biggest stressors in remote settings is being the person on the ground when the specialist is not available.

Support means predictable access to consultation:

- Scheduled case rounds (even brief, consistent)
- A clear process for urgent clinical questions
- Rapid consult pathways for acute risk decisions
- Shared protocols for common crises (withdrawal, psychosis, suicidality, agitation)

Staff tolerate hardship better when they know they are not alone.

2) *Training That Is Practical And Local*

Training in the North works best when it is:

- Short, repeated, and scenario-based
- Tailored to the actual local cases (breaches, intoxication, trauma, psychosis, cognitive decline, domestic violence)
- Designed for mixed teams (health and justice together)
- Grounded in what staff can realistically do with available resources

The goal is not to turn everyone into a specialist. The goal is to strengthen "first responses" and reduce the helpless feeling that drives burnout.

3) *Emotional Support Without Stigma*

Northern staff often carry vicarious trauma and moral injury. They witness suffering in a small community where they cannot "go home and forget." They see the same people in crisis again and again. They may know the families personally.

Support means:

- Regular debriefing structures after serious incidents
- Access to confidential counselling without career penalty
- Leadership that normalizes stress reactions as human, not weak
- Protected time for reflection, supervision, and learning

In systems where toughness is prized, emotional support must be framed as professionalism, not therapy.

4) *Respect For Local Intelligence*

Retention is improved when local staff are treated as experts in their environment, not as "helpers" to southern specialists.

Local teams know:

- Which plans are fantasy
- Which families can support safely
- Which conditions will predictably fail
- Which cultural pathways actually hold trust
- What the community will accept and what will backfire

When visiting professionals collaborate humbly with that knowledge, staff feel valued, and the system becomes smarter.

VISITING MODELS THAT BUILD CAPACITY RATHER THAN DEPENDENCY

Visiting models can either strengthen local capacity or unintentionally weaken it.

A dependency model looks like this:

- Visiting specialist arrives
- Takes over the hardest cases
- Produces recommendations
- Leaves
- Local staff are left holding an unworkable plan
- The system waits for the next visit

- Local confidence erodes and frustration grows

A capacity-building model looks different.

1) *Co-Assessment And Co-Formulation*

Instead of the visitor doing the assessment alone, the visitor works alongside local staff:

- Sharing reasoning in real time
- Explaining formulation and risk logic
- Inviting local correction of assumptions
- Documenting in a way that local staff can use after the visitor leaves

This turns each visit into training without requiring a separate training day.

2) *Shared-Care Pathways With Clear Roles*

Capacity-building visits clarify who does what:

- The visiting psychiatrist handles forensic questions, diagnostic complexity, and medication strategy
- Local staff handle continuity, daily monitoring, cultural anchoring, and follow-up logistics
- Both share a common plan with contingency steps

The plan must be written for the people who stay, not the person who leaves.

3) *"Teach-Back" To The System, Not Just The Patient*

We often use teach-back with patients: "Tell me what you understood." Capacity-building uses teach-back with teams:

- "What part of this plan feels realistic?"
- "Where will it fail?"
- "What should we simplify?"
- "Who is the point person?"
- "What do we do if the flight cancels and we cannot transfer?"

This respects local staff as co-designers, not implementers of someone else's idea.

4) *Tele-Forensics As Continuity, Not Replacement*

Tele-forensics can either create dependency ("call the specialist for everything") or create strength ("use the specialist to support local decision-making").

The difference is design:

- Scheduled case conferences
- Clear thresholds for escalation
- Shared protocols
- Mentorship and supervision components
- Documentation templates that local staff can maintain

The goal is to make local staff more confident over time, not less.

5) *Build "Locals As Trainers"*

The most sustainable model is when northern staff become the trainers for their own region, supported by visiting expertise when needed.

That requires:

- Train-the-trainer approaches
- Protected time for leadership and teaching
- Recognition and career pathways that make staying professionally meaningful
- Compensation structures that match responsibility

People stay longer when they can grow.

RETENTION IS ALSO ABOUT DIGNITY

There is a blunt truth: many retention efforts fail because they treat the North as a hardship posting rather than a place where professionals can build a respected career.

Retention improves when staff experience:

- Adequate housing and safety
- Manageable workloads
- Time off that is real
- Professional development that is accessible
- Leadership that listens
- Respect from visiting specialists rather than being treated as "support staff"

- A sense that the system is improving, not only surviving

People can tolerate difficulty. What they cannot tolerate for long is futility.

WHAT I CAME TO BELIEVE

The Arctic does not need more visiting heroes. It needs visiting models that make themselves less necessary over time.

That is the paradox: the best visiting service is the one that leaves behind stronger local capacity each year, until "specialist scarcity" feels less like a crisis and more like a manageable reality.

Training and retention are not side issues. They are the foundation of safety, clinical safety, legal safety, and community safety.

Because in the end, the most reliable care is not the care that flies in.

It is the care that is already there, supported well enough to stay.

CHAPTER 33

Leaving Well

The hotel clock crawled toward 2:00 a.m., and sleep refused to arrive. My bag was half-zipped. The boarding pass was folded into the passport. My notes were stacked in an order that felt sensible at the time and would almost certainly feel absurd a week later. Outside, the entire community had gone quiet in that northern way: radiator ticking, hallway asleep, darkness settled like a second blanket.

Ottawa was waiting. But so was the familiar ache of circuit work: the excitement of going home braided with the discomfort of leaving.

Rankin Inlet had become, quickly and without ceremony, like a home. Not because I belonged there in any permanent sense—I did not—but because the North has a way of doing this: it lets you in through ordinary acts rather than grand welcomes. A multi-passenger taxi ride where strangers become temporary companions. Familiar faces in a hotel lobby. A greeting that is warm without being intrusive.

And then, unexpectedly, a table.

A local teacher, I will call her Ms. A, had invited me into her home. She had children with the bright, unfiltered honesty that makes adults remember what sincerity sounds like. That first evening, the smell arrived before the words: something rich simmering on the stove.

Caribou stew.

I had once sworn off caribou after an early trip to Iqaluit. One bad experience had lodged itself into memory as a permanent "never again." But vows about food are often vows about control, and the North does not always let you keep them. Ms. A served the stew without drama, no speech, no insistence, just a bowl placed in front of me like an invitation.

We ate, and the evening unfolded gently, stories moving back and forth, laughter appearing without force, cultural anecdotes bridging differences without making them a spectacle. Ms. A spoke about her classroom, about the community shifting quietly, about newcomers arriving and the choice to make welcome something practical rather than symbolic. She had noticed more African Canadian families and decided, simply, that "settling in" should mean belonging. She had organized small events, nothing grand, just enough to say: we see you, we want you here, your stories belong among ours.

The next day, she helped coordinate a mental health education session with children. Standing in front of those young faces, I heard my own children's advice in my head: keep it simple, honest, fun, and felt the tenderness of it. Children reward sincerity. They lean toward clarity. They ask what adults circle around. They remind you that good communication often sounds like humility.

By early morning, Ms. A drove me to the airport. Her children giggled in the back seat, laughter puncturing the quiet like small bells. The terminal was small and intimate, less a transit point than a community room with security gates. I thanked her, inadequate words for what I meant. She smiled and said something simple that landed like a fact: "You are welcome here."

When the plane lifted off, Rankin Inlet fell away beneath the wings: white, blue, vast. I watched until the buildings became points, and the points dissolved into distance.

The plane always leaves.

And that is exactly why leaving well matters.

Leaving is part of the job. But leaving well is a skill, one with ethical weight. In circuit work, your departure is not a neutral ending. It is a moment when plans either hold or collapse, when local staff either inherit clarity or inherit confusion, when a person either feels anchored by a realistic pathway or abandoned with a document that cannot be lived.

In southern practice, continuity is built into the environment. You hand over to a colleague down the hall. The chart stays in one hospital. The patient can return next week. The plan can be adjusted when it fails.

On circuit, none of that is guaranteed. Discontinuity is designed into the model. Specialists arrive, assess, write, testify, and depart. The system moves on. The weather overrules. The next docket begins.

So, leaving well becomes part of competence.

HANDOVERS THAT TRANSFER RESPONSIBILITY, NOT JUST INFORMATION

A handover is not a summary. It is a transfer of responsibility.

The most harmful handovers are the ones that look complete but are not usable: elegant formulations with no operational steps, long histories with no clear next action, recommendations that assume resources that do not exist, "follow up as needed" written into a place where "as needed" can mean "never."

Leaving well means designing handovers for the people who stay.

In the North, I learned to judge the quality of a plan with one blunt test:

WHAT HAPPENS ON THURSDAY NIGHT?

Not in theory. In practice. When the clinic is closed, when the phone is dead, when conflict rises in an overcrowded house, when cravings spike, when someone becomes paranoid, when the only open door is the nursing station or the jail.

A good handover includes:

- Clear triggers and early warning signs (what to look for before escalation becomes crisis)
- Concrete de-escalation strategies that local staff can actually use
- One identified point person (a name, not "the team")
- If/then contingencies for predictable failures (missed appointments, relapse, housing collapse, flight cancellations)
- Medication plans that match local formularies and monitoring capacity
- Victim-safety considerations that are realistic in small communities where anonymity is impossible

It also includes something the system often avoids: limits.

If the assessment was constrained by time, language, missing collateral, fluctuating symptoms, or environmental effects of remand, that must be named plainly. Not to protect the clinician's ego, but to protect everyone downstream from false certainty.

FOLLOW-UP PLANS THAT ARE REAL, NOT PERFORMATIVE

In the Arctic, "follow-up" can become a ritual phrase, written because it sounds responsible, not because it will happen.

Leaving well means resisting the temptation to recommend ideal pathways that will collapse on contact with local reality. If a service is intermittent or absent, do not write as if it is routine. If appointments depend on flights, say so. If the plan depends on stable housing that does not exist, name the gap.

A realistic follow-up plan begins with the first week after release, often the highest-risk window, and makes it concrete:

- Where will the person sleep tonight?
- Who will check in within 24–72 hours?
- What is the plan for sleep restoration?
- What is the relapse response that reduces harm rather than producing automatic breach?
- What does the person do if they begin to escalate at night?

Then it builds a ladder:

- Best case: scheduled follow-up occurs.
- If disrupted: phone contact or in-person check with local staff.
- If crisis: nursing station or emergency pathway.
- If safety threat: immediate steps to protect victims and prevent escalation.

This is not over-planning. It is designing for interruption because interruption is normal.

DOCUMENTATION THAT HELPS RATHER THAN HARMS

Forensic documentation can stabilize a case or distort it for years.

In small communities, a phrase travels. A label sticks. A careless sentence can become a reputation.

Leaving well means writing with disciplined humility:

- Be specific, not global. Replace moral adjectives ("manipulative," "noncompliant," "bad insight") with observable patterns and plausible mechanisms.
- Separate facts, observations, and inferences. What the person said. What records show. What you observed. What you infer, and why. What remains uncertain.
- Avoid "paper safety." Don't recommend conditions that look protective but are unlivable: curfews without safe housing, abstinence without treatment access, no-contact orders without realistic avoidance strategies in a small place.
- Don't build breach traps. If a condition is likely to fail because of cognitive limitations, trauma-driven dysregulation, addiction, or scarcity, either simplify it or explicitly recommend supports that make compliance possible. A report should never function as a quiet machine for manufacturing breaches.

ENDING THE CIRCUIT WITHOUT ABANDONING THE PEOPLE IN IT

You cannot change one truth: people feel your departure. Some are indifferent. Some are angry. Some are quietly hopeful. Some feel exposed by what was assessed and then left to carry it alone. Local staff, who remain, carry the real continuity burden after you leave.

So, leaving well requires closing loops:

- Ensure local staff have what they need while you are still reachable.
- Clarify who owns follow-up for urgent cases.
- Reduce ambiguity, because ambiguity becomes burden.

- Where appropriate, ensure the person assessed understands, in plain language, what happens next procedurally, without promising outcomes you cannot control.

Leaving well is not about staying forever. It is about departing with care.

THE RULE I TRIED TO LIVE BY

Over time, I developed a private rule, simple, unforgiving, and useful:

Don't leave behind a plan you would not want to inherit.

Not if you were the nurse on night shift.

Not if you were the court worker explaining conditions in plain language.

Not if you were the probation officer trying to make compliance possible.

Not if you were the family member holding the person together after release.

If the plan depends on resources that are not there, rewrite it.

If the plan requires perfect compliance from a chaotic life, simplify it.

If the plan collapses when the flight cancels, add contingencies.

If the language stigmatizes, make it precise and human.

Because the plane will always leave.

And what remains, after the engines fade and the runway becomes a line in the snow, is whatever you left behind: your words, your recommendations, your handover, your clarity or confusion.

The North taught me that departure is not the end of the work. It is part of the work.

Leaving well is how a visitor honors the people who stay.

Afterword

WHAT THE ARCTIC TAUGHT ME ABOUT JUSTICE, HEALING, AND HUMILITY

The Arctic taught me that justice is not only what happens in court.

Justice is what happens after court, on the walk home, in the crowded house, in the quiet hours when cravings rise, in the long nights when fear returns, in the moment a person decides whether to call for help or to disappear. The courtroom can pronounce an outcome, but the land decides what that outcome can realistically become.

At first, I arrived with the habits of southern practice: confidence in systems, faith in referrals, comfort with neat categories. Over time, the North stripped those comforts away. The North demanded precision without arrogance, compassion without rescue fantasies, and recommendations that could survive the blunt truth of distance.

I learned that a "reasonable condition" can be impossible. That a breach can be predictable. That remand can be geography disguised as accountability. That a plane ticket can be a treatment plan and a rupture at the same time. That a phone call can be the only bridge for hundreds of kilometers, and that bridges fail.

I learned, too, that healing is not a single intervention. It is a chain. In remote places, the chain breaks easily, and the person gets blamed for falling when the truth is simpler: there was nothing to hold onto.

And I learned humility in a more embodied way than any lecture ever offered. Humility is not a posture. It is a practice: listening more than speaking, checking assumptions, respecting silence, accepting that community knowledge often outruns my credentials. It is understanding that

I am a visitor, one voice among many, and that the people who keep the system alive are the ones who stay when the plane leaves.

The Arctic also taught me that people are not reducible to their worst day.

The young person with too many breaches was not a file; he was a nervous system raised on scarcity and chaos. The woman on remand was not a charge; she was a mother trying to survive coercion and shame while separated from her children. The Elder was not "difficult"; he was confused, vulnerable, and proud, misread by a system built for faster minds. Even the man everyone feared was not a myth; he was a predictable outcome of escalating violence and missed early intervention, carrying shame that turned outward because it had nowhere safe to go.

None of this erases harm. Victims are real. Fear is real. Accountability is real. But the North taught me that safety is not achieved by paperwork alone. Safety is achieved by plans that can be lived, supports that can be reached, and systems that can hold people long enough for change to become more than a promise spoken in court.

If this book has one message, it is not that the Arctic is tragic or heroic. It is that the Arctic is honest. It does not tolerate pretend solutions. It forces every system—justice, health, social services—to confront its own limits without excuses.

And still, it also offers a quiet kind of hope: that better is possible, not through grand declarations, but through continuity, cultural safety, practical design, and the humility to build with communities rather than for them.

The plane always leaves.

But what the Arctic taught me is that leaving does not have to mean abandoning, if we learn how to hand over well, how to write responsibly, how to train and retain, and how to build justice and care that fit the land and the lives lived on it.

That is the work.

And it is work worth returning to.

Suggested Reading and Resources

Forensic Psychiatry and Law (Canada-focused where possible)

- *Criminal Code of Canada*, Part XX.1 (Mental Disorder) and related provisions for NCRMD/fitness frameworks.
- *Winko v. British Columbia (Forensic Psychiatric Institute)* (Supreme Court of Canada), foundational decision on NCRMD dispositions and balancing public safety.
- *R. v. Swain* and subsequent SCC jurisprudence shaping Part XX.1 principles.
- Canadian Academy of Psychiatry and the Law (CAPL), position statements, educational resources, and conference proceedings; useful for Canadian practice norms.
- Royal College of Physicians and Surgeons of Canada, CanMEDS framework and psychiatry competencies relevant to forensic practice.

Risk Assessment and Violence Prevention (general evidence base)

- Structured professional judgment tools and manuals commonly used in forensic settings (e.g., HCR-20 for violence risk, START for short-term risk).
- Core literature on risk formulation and management principles, emphasizing dynamic risk, protective factors, and scenario-based planning.

Trauma-Informed Justice and Coercive Control

- Foundational trauma-informed care frameworks emphasizing safety, trust, choice, collaboration, and empowerment.
- Evidence and policy resources on intimate partner violence, coercive control, and intersections with criminalization and remand.

Northern and Indigenous Health, Cultural Safety

- Truth and Reconciliation Commission of Canada (TRC) Calls to Action relevant to health and justice.
- National Inquiry into Missing and Murdered Indigenous Women and Girls (MMIWG) Calls for Justice, focusing on health and justice intersections.
- Health Canada and Indigenous Services Canada resources on Indigenous health and culturally safe service delivery.
- Cultural safety training materials endorsed by provincial or territorial health authorities and Indigenous-led organizations.

Arctic/Northern Mental Health Systems and Service Design

- Policy and planning documents from territorial health authorities (Nunavut, NWT, Yukon) regarding mental health, addictions, and suicide prevention.
- Literature on tele-mental health, rural and remote service delivery, and continuity-of-care models.

Practical, Local-Facing Resources (reader-oriented)

- Crisis line information relevant to northern Canada (territorial and national).
- Patient-facing resources on trauma, substance use, sleep, and coping skills that are accessible, culturally respectful, and non-stigmatizing.

www.ingramcontent.com/pod-product-compliance
Lightning Source LLC
Chambersburg PA
CBHW031322230926
51848CB00001B/48